Praise for Roy Taylor's *Li.*

'Fascinating, informative and, in today's world,
important. For anyone with type 2 diabetes, it's a
no-brainer – follow Roy's roadmap and reverse it.
And if you haven't got type 2 diabetes – yet –
follow Roy's roadmap and avoid it.'
Jimmy Nail

'Roy Taylor and his team at Newcastle University have
not only cracked the mystery of what causes type 2
diabetes, the greatest health problem of our time, but
shown the world how to get rid of it. This is a terrific
book, which will help a huge number of people.'
Dr Michael Mosley

'Professor Taylor's remarkable tenacity in researching
the concept that some people are able to put their type 2
diabetes into remission is changing how we think about
and treat this pervasive condition.'
Elizabeth Robertson,
Director of Research, Diabetes UK

'This fine book contains good science, good writing
and good advice in equal measure. It is both
fascinating and useful for readers.'
Matt Ridley,
author of *The Evolution of Everything*

Your simple guide to
REVERSING
TYPE 2
DIABETES

Your simple guide to
REVERSING
TYPE 2
DIABETES

Professor Roy Taylor

Professor of Medicine and Metabolism,
Newcastle University
and
Honorary Consultant Physician
Newcastle upon Tyne Hospitals
NHS Foundation Trust

Published in 2021 by Short Books,
an imprint of Octopus Publishing Group Ltd
Carmelite House, 50 Victoria Embankment
London, EC4Y 0DZ
www.octopusbooks.co.uk
www.shortbooks.co.uk

An Hachette UK Company
www.hachette.co.uk

10 9

A CIP catalogue record for this book is available from the British Library.

ISBN: 978-1-78072-499-7

Cover design by Andrew Smith

Printed and bound in Great Britain by Clays Ltd, Elcograf S.p.A.

This FSC® label means that materials used for the
product have been responsibly sourced.

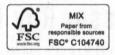

The author will donate 100% of his proceeds from this
book to Diabetes UK (a registered charity in England
and Wales (no 215199) and Scotland (SC039136)).
This is expected to be at least £15,000.

In aid of

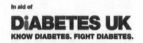

*This book is dedicated to my patients and research volunteers, who **have** taught me so much*

This is a book for everyone. Do you have type 2 diabetes? Pre-diabetes? Do you have type 2 diabetes in your family? Do you feel at risk? Perhaps you want to reduce your risk of getting seriously ill – including with Coronavirus. Maybe you are just curious about type 2 diabetes and want to know the real facts about it. In that case, read on!

Contents

Part I

WHAT IS TYPE 2 DIABETES?

Chapter 1

What causes type 2 diabetes?

Put simply, 'diabetes' just means the level of sugar in the blood is too high.

In healthy people, blood sugar levels are kept very steady. In people with type 2 diabetes, blood sugar levels are too high overnight and even higher after eating.

Does this matter? Sugar looks so innocent, sitting there in the sugar bowl. It can be added to almost everything – from a cup of tea to burgers. But, yes, it does matter, because high sugar levels in the blood can cause problems throughout the body.

This book is all about type 2 diabetes, the commonest form of the disease – 9 out of 10 people with diabetes will have this type. It is very different from type 1 diabetes which typically develops in children and younger adults. There are also other types of diabetes but these are much less common. All types result in high blood sugar levels, and can cause serious health problems. Being completely sure that a person has true type 2 diabetes is sometimes tricky. But if you are over 30 years old, and have put on weight in adult life, and have high blood sugars, it is very likely that you have type 2 diabetes.

The Covid-19 pandemic has brought diabetes into the headlines because it makes serious illness – or worse – much more likely. As if diabetes was not bad enough already.

If you or someone close to you has type 2 diabetes, you will probably have a lot of questions. Just why can't my body keep sugar levels normal? What will diabetes do to me? Is it the serious kind? What actually causes type 2 diabetes? Let's look at some of these questions in turn.

Why do sugar levels shoot up after meals?

As soon as you take your first mouthful of any food, your body starts to break it down. All the starchy food is turned into sugar and that rapidly gets into the blood. For instance, from an ordinary helping of pasta, about 30 teaspoonfuls of sugar are released. 30 spoonfuls!

Your body will get almost the same effect from eating the pasta or the sugar, except for slight differences in the speed at which it gets into the blood. To deal with this sudden rush of sugar, your pancreas normally makes lots of insulin, which allows the body to use the sugar or store it away. But in type 2 diabetes this does not happen and so blood sugar levels rise rapidly.

This is the major problem of diabetes. It is the failure to make enough insulin at the right time.

To make matters worse, even the insulin your pancreas does make does not work so well. This is called 'insulin resistance'. It means that your body does not respond well to whatever insulin is on offer.

But why is my sugar level high even when I haven't been eating?

If you have diabetes, you may be puzzled to find that your blood sugar is high even first thing in the morning – when you have not eaten anything for 12 hours or more. Sometimes it can be even higher early in the morning than it was at bed time. What is going on? Surely you didn't raid the fridge overnight?

To explain this, I need to tell you about the neat way that blood sugar is normally controlled overnight. First thing in the morning, none of the sugar in your blood is from food. In fact, all of it has been made by your own body – by your liver. Why does your body make this dangerous stuff? Well, because a constant level of sugar is vital to fuel your body. All parts of your body need a constant supply of energy. So your liver normally makes just the right amount. Day and night.

In type 2 diabetes, however, your liver is making too much sugar and has nowhere to store it so keeps pumping it out into your bloodstream.

What are the immediate problems of type 2 diabetes?

Diabetes might be discovered during routine testing. But, if your diabetes was diagnosed because you had troublesome symptoms, then you will already know about some of the problems it can cause.

When blood sugar levels go too high, sugar spills over into the urine. And, because sugar draws water along with it, this causes the kidneys to make more urine than usual. Passing too much urine is a sure sign that blood sugar has become too high. If your diabetes gets badly out of control – perhaps if you have eaten too much or if you have forgotten to take your tablets or injections – you are likely to find that you have to get up in the night to go to the loo more often. And because water is being lost from the body, you will feel thirsty.

Other problems may have occurred early on:

- Feeling generally tired and out of sorts
- Infections of the skin, most commonly of the penis or vulva causing itching and redness
- Foot problems including discoloured toes (this can happen early on because diabetes can be causing damage for a long time before it is diagnosed).

Skin infections tend to be due to candida infections, but any sort of infection is more likely when blood sugar levels are raised. Breaks in the skin – small cuts or other trivial injuries – are prone to get infected, and urine infections are very common, too. This may sound like a depressing list – but these issues are not the worst of it.

And the long-term problems?

I have just described the immediate effects of blood sugar being too high. If blood sugar levels are raised for years, then more serious long-term problems will start stacking up.

Left too high for years, raised sugar levels can damage the delicate blood vessels that supply food and oxygen to all parts of the body. When organs don't get their regular grocery order, they stop working properly.

The eye is particularly sensitive. The back of your eye can become damaged, threatening your eyesight. Tragically, diabetes is a common cause of loss of vision. Before effective eye screening was developed, it was the commonest preventable cause of blindness in the UK.

Nerves anywhere in the body can be damaged. Have you ever experienced a 'dead-leg'? By sitting awkwardly and squeezing a nerve for too long you can block capillary flow of blood to the nerve and cause it to stop working. If you are in normal health, the numbness and not being able to walk properly will go away within a few minutes of relieving the pressure. But nerve problems in diabetes are not so easily reversed, because they result from years of damage to those tiny blood vessels which keep nerves working. Numbness, tingling and even pain can last for months and may become permanent.

Numbness in feet is a particular problem because it prevents the body's normal warning sign of trouble – i.e. pain. If your new shoes are rubbing, of course you will stop walking or change shoes. But if you cannot feel the pain you will carry on walking while the damage continues silently. This can lead to skin breaking down and opens the door to infections possibly with devastating consequences. In diabetes, the motto for feet is 'Check 'em or lose 'em'. This may sound brutal, but there is no point in my putting a gloss on things here: providing clear information about the very real risks is essential. You do not want a doctor who will cover up the hard truth. In the UK today about 170 amputations are performed every week because of diabetes. Yes, *every week*.

High sugar levels can also cause the kidneys not just to struggle but to lose function altogether. Diabetes accounts for around half of patients needing kidney dialysis treatment. This has to be done three times every week, and it severely affects enjoyment of life.

Unfortunately, the problems caused by diabetes do not end there. It can bring about fatty changes to blood vessel walls, so that they become more easily blocked. Blockages in the blood vessels to the heart muscle cause heart attacks. Blockages in those supplying the brain cause strokes. This is why heart attacks and strokes are much commoner in people with diabetes. Blockages in the main blood vessels to the legs cause poor circulation to the feet making other problems worse, and amputation more likely.

Your risk factor for developing any of these problems depends quite a lot on the age when diabetes starts. Unlike certain other illnesses where your youth may be on your side, type 2 diabetes puts people in their twenties or thirties at far greater risk of serious trouble. The younger you are, the worse the effects of type 2 diabetes.

- Young people getting type 2 diabetes will suffer worse health problems even than those getting type 1 diabetes, the kind that requires insulin injections right from the start.

- A 45-year-old man newly diagnosed with diabetes has a more than a 50% chance of having to stop work and retire early because of heart attacks, stroke or serious foot problems. That 45- year-old-man will lose an average of six years of life.

- But for anyone who is diagnosed at the age of 70 years or over, the chance of major health problems remains the same as someone of the same age without diabetes.

Is Covid-19 worse if you have type 2 diabetes?

If you have diabetes you are much more likely to become severely ill with Covid-19. You are also at greater risk of dying from it – *almost seven times* more likely, according to the largest study conducted so far.

This figure was so high because type 2 diabetes is commoner in older people, and older people are more likely to die with Covid-19. But, even after accounting for age and weight, if you have diabetes you are more than twice as likely to die with Covid than a similar person who does not have diabetes. That is a grim fact.

But you can take positive action and get back to normal health, as this book shows. If you are carrying too much weight, your chances of getting severe Covid-19, and of dying of it, will certainly be decreased if you severely cut back on the amount of food you eat.

Likewise, if you have type 2 diabetes, and you want to reduce your risk of becoming seriously ill or even dying, you need to lose a significant amount of weight. As well as avoiding the misery of living with the usual threats from type 2 – premature heart attack and stroke, loss of eyesight, loss of limb and the burden of medication – you will reduce your chances of succumbing to all sorts of other nasty conditions. Many types of cancers happen more commonly in people with type 2 diabetes. Likewise, some very unpleasant infections are commoner in diabetes, and although rare they can ruin life.

What causes type 2 diabetes?

Type 2 diabetes just does not happen when food is scarce. When poverty or wars cause a population to be suddenly short of food, the number of people with type 2 diabetes drops sharply. This occurred during both world wars.

Famously, in a study done around 1900, one group of Native American people was found to have no cases at all. The Pima Indians were successful farmers in a barren part of Arizona, growing just enough food to eat. Today they have the highest incidence of type 2 diabetes in the world – about one in two adults have the condition. What happened was that they were displaced from their lands, and thus forced to stop farming. This had a significant effect on their levels of physical activity and the food they ate. Rather than growing their own, they were given hand-outs. This is a dramatic story, and it illustrates an important fact: even people who are genetically suscep-tible do not get type 2 diabetes unless they eat more food than they actually need. What the genes do is to increase the chance of excess fat causing type 2 diabetes. But, no matter what one's genes, the fact is stark – no excess fat no diabetes.

I am not obese so why do I have type 2 diabetes?

Whatever you may read in the headlines, type 2 diabetes has very little to do with obesity. The words 'obese' and 'obesity' are often used thoughtlessly. In medical terms, obesity is defined as having a body mass index of greater than 30. And according to this definition, for every two people developing type 2 diabetes only one will be 'obese'. What is true is that everyone with type 2 diabetes is carrying more weight *than their own body can cope with*.

The trouble is that many people regard themselves as having a normal weight because they look similar to the most other people of the same age. But that is not necessarily healthy.

Are you the same weight as you were when you were 25 years old? Just look at folk in the high street: people aged in their twenties tend to be slimmer than those in their sixties. In Britain and similar societies, we gain around a pound in weight each year through most of our adult life. There is no biological reason, however, why people need to put on weight during adult life. Putting weight on has nothing to do with ageing or with hormones – it simply reflects the environment we live in.

And that environment is setting up a time bomb. In the UK, over one third of people start adult life far too heavy, and those who are susceptible to type 2 diabetes are sure to develop the disease at a younger age than their parents. This time bomb deserves a book to itself.

What is pre-diabetes?

Type 2 diabetes does not come on suddenly. It creeps up on you over many years. And during that time your blood sugar will be slowly rising. At some point, your doctor may tell you that it is a bit on the high side. That is pre-diabetes: the grey zone when your blood sugar is higher than ideal.

After a few more years, with no changes in your life-style, your blood sugar is likely to get even higher – but may still be in that grey zone. And then comes the day when you doctor says 'You have diabetes'.

Diabetes is bad news – but so is pre-diabetes.

If you have pre-diabetes then you are at much greater risk of heart attacks and strokes. The reason is simple: these terrible illnesses are caused by the same thing that is causing the slow development of type 2 diabetes: more fat inside your body than you can cope with. I will explain how our individual fat thresholds affect our risk of diabetes in the Chapter 4, but the important thing to emphasise here is that a blood sugar which is on the high side needs action. Fortunately, pre-diabetes is easier to reverse than type 2 diabetes. But be under no illusions: the writing is on the wall. Your health is under serious threat.

Quick read

- 'Diabetes' means that your blood sugar is too high

- It is caused by the pancreas not making insulin fast enough

- Furthermore, what insulin your body does make does not work properly

- Immediate problems include thirst, passing too much urine and tiredness

- Pre-diabetes means that your health is already damaged and you need to take action

- The long-term complications of diabetes can be very serious

Chapter 2

The 'usual' treatment for type 2 diabetes

Today's usual treatment for type 2 diabetes is not great. Although I discovered that it could be reversed to normal back in 2011, the guidelines for primary care have yet to be fully updated, and so many doctors are still treating the condition in the old way. It takes a long time for new discoveries to be accepted in medical practice.

In this chapter, I'm going to describe what the conventional guidelines say is in store for you if you have type 2. That is the bad news often handed out at diagnosis. The good news is that the rest of this book tells you how to avoid this fate.

The conventional guidelines describe a depressing future: lifelong diabetes. You must learn to live with it, taking steadily increasing numbers of tablets, then going on to injections, then insulin treatment. If you are newly diagnosed with type 2 diabetes you may be told that you have a 50:50 chance of being on insulin injections within ten years.

You may also be told that you should lose weight and take more exercise. But, this advice is usually given casually and without any clear information as to how to go about it. You may get the impression that your doctor or nurse does not think weight loss is likely to be achievable. You may be given a 'diet sheet' – even though we know that diet sheets by themselves are ineffective.

Tablets

But most often, the immediate step after diagnosis is to be prescribed a tablet to help keep your blood sugar down. This will usually be 'metformin'. Metformin is a cheap drug that comes in the size of a horse pill and has several side effects.

Some of these side effects can be troubling. In quite a few people it causes tummy discomfort and loose bowels. But remember that, from the point of view of a doctor or nurse, the most important thing is whether a tablet has the desired effect – of controlling your blood sugar. The term 'side effects' is therefore often used as a way of describing things that are troubling to you rather than to the person who is treating you. Perhaps we should change these medical words, and talk about the *total effects* of a drug – after all, you are the expert on what is happening to your body. Tablets can be very useful, but they do have drawbacks.

One good thing about metformin is that it does not cause you to put on more weight. It is also a relatively safe drug in most people. But metformin has only a modest effect on blood sugar control and after a while other tablets have to be added in. The cheaper options all cause weight gain and can cause you to become suddenly dizzy if your sugar levels drop too low. The medicines that can cause low blood sugar attacks – 'hypos' – include gliclazide, glibenclamide and gliquidone. Others do not cause hypos, but pile on the weight, or can make your ankles swell. The most expensive newer options (gliptins or gliflozins) do neither of these things but have other 'side effects'.

Injections

Over time you may have to take two or three different tablets and if your sugar levels are still uncontrolled, other medicines may be recommended such as exenatide (or Byetta) and liraglutide (or Victoza). These have to be injected and are at present expensive and not widely used.

These medicines slow down stomach-emptying after a meal, and stop food from getting into the body too fast; which in turn slows down the rise in blood sugar after eating. They also have the really useful effect of limiting the amount of food you eat, as the stomach stays full for longer. They do cause some weight loss – but only a few pounds. Some people feel a bit nauseous when they start this treatment – but don't worry, it is only a 'side effect'!

Insulin injections

And then there is insulin. In many people who have had type 2 diabetes for a long time, insulin can improve the control of blood sugar, but the devil is in the detail of its 'side effects'. Insulin usually causes your weight to increase. That is not welcome. It can also cause low blood sugar attacks. These hypos can cause all kinds of problems in day-to-day life – for instance when driving, climbing up ladders, or just simply pottering around the kitchen.

What do you mean by 'treatable', doctor?

If you were to ask 'Can my diabetes be treated, doctor?' they would say, 'Yes'. But the doctor may not be answering the question as you intended it. There are official guidelines on how type 2 diabetes should be treated, and certainly a range of treatment options are available. The real meaning of your question may have been: can treatment bring my body back to normal, in the same way that antibiotics do when you have an infection, or an op does if you have appendicitis?

The reply that type 2 diabetes can be 'treated' conveys the wrong message to many people and may give a false sense of security. Worse still, well-meaning government or charity information sites tend to make light of the problems caused by diabetes. They give the impression that life can continue pretty much as normal. The hard truth is not stated – that the main problems of diabetes are only slightly improved by treatment, and that there is still a high risk of ill health as a result.

Food for diabetes or diabetic food?

In chemists and supermarkets you may see shelves labelled 'diabetic foods'. Avoid them: they contain at least as many calories as their ordinary varieties of the same products. They do not make a worthwhile difference to blood sugar control and certainly do not help with weight loss. All doctors and health professionals discourage the use of 'diabetic foods', because they do simply not help.

It is far more effective to cut back on both sugar and your total consumption of food and alcohol than to opt for special foods. For instance, halving your portion of potato/pasta/rice and doubling your serving of vegetables would be good. There are plenty more ideas later in the book about how to set in place better eating habits.

Annual checks

Management of diabetes is not all bad news. One of the triumphs of modern diabetes care in the UK (and some other countries) is that the main curse of the disease has been lifted. When I was appointed as a consultant in 1985, there were six people under the age of 25 years in my clinic who were already registered as blind due to diabetes. Today there are none, largely because annual checks using a simple, effective test have become part of routine healthcare in the UK. If picked up early enough, deterioration can be prevented by specialist eye treatment.

Also, regular checking of blood pressure for diabetes patients has led to early treatment being widely advised. It is straightforward to reduce a person's blood pressure using tablets. And active treatment of blood pressure has a big effect, in particular, on decreasing the chance of kidney failure and strokes. A simple annual urine test gives a good early warning of any trouble.

Regular checking of feet can also detect early problems and avoid trouble. Feet tend to be the most neglected part of the body and are the butt of comedian's jokes. But your feet are amazing works of engineering which you may not notice until you lose one. Your feet are well worth checking. Well worth looking after. So take off your shoes and have a good inspection at least once a year!

All the measures mentioned above can help 'manage' the symptoms of type 2 diabetes, and these annual checks can be successful in decreasing serious problems for people with the disease, but how much better it would be to prevent any such problems occurring at all – by reversing your diabetes altogether. You have a choice – accept pills, potions and problems *or* make a bid to return to full health.

Quick read

- Tablet treatment can decrease blood sugar a little
- It does not stop the steady worsening of sugar levels
- Tablets can cause unpleasant side effects

- Insulin treatment is needed by one person in two within ten years of diagnosis
- An annual diabetes check is a vital part of treatment as it helps lower the risk of bad complications

Part II

WHY WE GET IT

Part II

WHY WE GET IT

Chapter 3

Why type 2 diabetes develops

Type 2 diabetes: let's call it food poisoning

Although we may think of poisons as being very different from other substances, it is really the amount swallowed that decides whether something is safe or poisonous. For instance, there are tiny traces of cyanide in apple pips but of course they are harmless to swallow. Even water can be bad for you – in large quantities. If you drink far too much water you may die. Similarly, vitamins are essential for life but in larger amounts some can be poisonous.

In just the same way, food is essential for life – but can be poisonous in excess. If you take just a little more than your own body needs every day *for a long time* you will run into problems. The most hazardous of these problems is type 2 diabetes.

The words 'food poisoning' usually make us think of tummy upsets caused by eating something bad. But in today's world they can be used to describe the long-term problems caused by eating too much food, year on year.

How does the body normally deal with food?

Food is used to fuel the body. And a healthy body is highly efficient at getting the most out of the food it receives.

After you finish a meal, the food you have eaten is stored away in order to provide a supply of sugar and fat. Energy from these stores is needed constantly, throughout the day and night. Every part of the body requires a steady supply of energy to keep functioning. And in normal health both of these processes – the storage of food and its later use – are tightly controlled.

This finely balanced system works very well, whatever you eat. Just think how differently people eat in different countries. Subsistence farmers in India live normal lives on a very high carbohydrate diet, while Innuits in the far north of Canada live normal lives on a very high fat diet. Humans can cope with a wide range of foods. The secret of how this happens lies in the amazing hormone insulin.

Insulin is made in the pancreas, an organ hidden deep behind your stomach. Quietly going about its business, it puts the right amount of insulin into the blood minute by minute. First, insulin travels from the pancreas via a special vein to the liver. Once there, it has the very important job of telling the liver how much sugar to release into the blood. The liver is constantly making sugar (from food previously eaten), to be carried by the blood to all parts of the body. It is thanks to insulin that the level of sugar in the blood usually stays in a narrow range whether you have just eaten or have just woken up after not eating for many hours. But in type 2 diabetes, the liver is no longer properly controlled by insulin and pours out far too much sugar into the blood.

How things may start to go wrong

Your remarkable body can cope with any mix of foods, but there is one thing that it may struggle with. And that is a little too much food too often over many years. It can be difficult to imagine what an extra tiny amount each day adds up to over the years, but, to give you an idea, an extra small apple every day, for instance, will add around four pounds to your weight in a year. Which means that ten years later you will be 40 pounds heavier! That is 2 stone 12 pounds (or 18kg). Surely that little apple cannot cause that? Yes it can!

If even a humble apple can make me put on weight,

you might ask – does it matter what I eat? Why should I bother making 'healthy' choices?

When it comes to the types of food you eat, there are three really important facts to know. All food is made up of fat, carbs and protein. And this is what happens when you eat them:

- If you eat more fat than your body needs, the excess gets stored as fat.

- If you eat more carbs than your body needs, the excess is converted into fat then stored.

- If you eat more protein than your body needs, the excess is converted into fat then stored.

So you see, whatever mix of foods you eat, anything *more than you need* simply gets stored as fat. A healthy diet is one that allows you to keep your weight at the right level for you.

That said, all foods are not equal. What you choose to eat does matter because certain types of food are more satisfying, and will keep you feeling full for longer, whereas others with the same calorie content are more rapidly absorbed by the body, after which you will quickly feel hungry again. So the type of food you eat affects the amount you eat overall. In the example above, it is easy to see that an additional two squares of milk chocolate (similar calorie count) are far more likely to slip down than an apple every single day. Similarly, if you eat a ready meal, which is likely to have lots of added sugar, you will probably feel hungry in an hour or so – and then you might eat more. On the other hand, a meal of meat and plenty of fibrous vegetables which has the same number of calories will leave you satisfied for much longer and stop you reaching out for a snack before your next meal.

There are huge commercial interests in selling diets that are labelled 'low fat' or 'low carbohydrate'. But the mix of foods is really only important as far as it suits you and helps you to avoid eating to excess in the long term.

When you eat more than your body needs, it has to find somewhere to store the extra fat. To begin with, fat will build up under the skin. It can be stored there safely – up to a point. But then it will start spilling over into the organs of the body, particularly the liver and the pancreas. And this is where it causes type 2 diabetes – in those people susceptible to it. Most people can tolerate too much fat in the pancreas, and never get type 2 diabetes. But if your pancreas happens to be less able to cope with fat, then you will run into trouble. It is the luck of the draw, depending on which genes you inherited.

Body weight during adult life

As I mentioned earlier, people in their twenties tend to be slimmer than those in their sixties, although there is no biological reason why we need to put on weight during adult life. It is also true to say that the average weight of the whole population has increased today. Of course there are some people who have changed from being heavy to being very heavy. But, with media attention focusing upon this serious obesity and showing pictures of very large people whenever type 2 diabetes is mentioned, you'd be forgiven for thinking that this was the main problem. Wrong! Even doctors sometimes state that the type 2 diabetes epidemic is 'due to obesity'. The effect of this misinformation is for a person to be accused of bringing the condition on themselves: 'Well, he's obese, it is all his own fault.' Wrong! Actually the problem is not the number of very, very heavy people. It is the vast majority who are just heavier than is ideal.

Body weight tends to remain much more stable in societies where food is not a heavily promoted pastime. That is particularly true if there is no way of getting around other than walking or cycling every day. But obviously, we live in a consumerist environment in the developed world, where enticing, quick-fix, carb-heavy food is everywhere and heavily marketed. You have to be unusually disciplined or just not that bothered by food to avoid putting on weight.

Not everyone who steadily puts on weight during their adult life will develop type 2 diabetes. Some people are much more susceptible to the disease than others. What is certain, though, is that if you have type 2 diabetes, your body will have had more food than it needed over many years. Your fat stores will be full to the brim. In fact, your body will be drowning in the excess food energy contained in the fat. Look at the text box below:

Why type 2 diabetes is caused by too much fat

1. Too much fat inside your liver stops insulin from working properly. That causes the liver to release too much sugar into the blood.

2. At the same time, too much fat inside your liver releases too much fat into your blood, fat which can't be safely stored away under the skin.

3. Excess fat from the blood seeps out everywhere in the body, including in your pancreas, with the result that the pancreas stops making insulin fast enough.

4. As a result, blood sugar levels will be high, especially after eating.

The crucial thing is that when it is clogged with excess fat your pancreas can no longer function properly. Even during the night when no food is being eaten, it will try to make insulin fast enough to control blood sugar levels but it won't quite manage. Then, after a meal, the problem gets much worse, when there is not enough insulin to cope with the sudden arrival of food in the body.

Fat and sugar are both vital in keeping you alive, but too much fat and sugar will poison your body. No wonder you may not feel at your best.

Type 2 diabetes takes at least ten years to develop in most people. The stores of fat build up very slowly – from eating too much of anything. If blood tests had been done a few years before you developed type 2 diabetes, your liver would have been sending out distress signals. In the years following, as you sped down the path to diagnosis, it was giving out a long, silent scream.

The secret life of the pancreas

The pancreas is a shy organ. It hides away and does its vital job of making insulin without fuss – normally. You never need to think about it, because it automatically makes the right amount of insulin whenever you need it.

Where exactly is it? Few people know, although they know perfectly well where their heart, their brain and their liver can be found. The pancreas lies partly behind and partly below your stomach. Put your hand over the front lower edge of your ribs on your left side. Your pancreas is deep inside, below your hand.

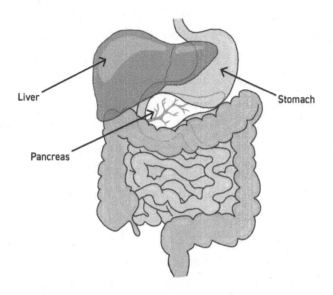

This picture shows where your pancreas lives. Imagine that the 'lid has been lifted off your abdomen – you are looking straight at your insides. The pancreas is behind your stomach, over on your left side.

The pancreas's position does not make it an easy organ to study. Brain specialists have a neatly packaged organ to focus upon, liver specialists have a big lump of an organ to examine, and heart specialists have a pump which is simple to test. The pancreas is a trickier customer. It is an odd-shaped, floppy organ, with one end butted against the start of the small intestine, and the other gradually tapering upwards to a small nub close to your ribs, far over on your left-hand side. It is tricky to scan not only because it is so deep inside but also because it is hidden in a layer of fat. As a result, the pancreas is the least studied organ in diabetes. Which is astonishing, given that it is the most important.

And then, to top it all, the pancreas does two main jobs, not one. Most of it is devoted to making the digestive juices that flow into the gut to break down the food we eat. This part comprises lots of tiny lobules which make the juices to be delivered to the intestine.

But none of this is about making insulin. Of the various hormones in our bodies, only a handful are vital for life. Insulin is one of them. Most hormones are made by a special gland – for instance, the thyroid gland in the neck, the adrenal gland above each kidney, or the ovaries and testes. Nothing so simple for our friend insulin, however! Insulin is made not by the whole pancreas, but by cells called beta cells, which are scattered throughout the organ.

Until recently, all that we knew about the human pancreas came from looking at it after death or after surgical removal because of disease. But now, thanks to special MRI scans, we know more about it than ever before. These scans led to the discoveries that this book is all about. They have enabled us to measure the level of fat within the pancreas itself and to examine its size and shape.

How big is your pancreas?

One day in 2014, one of my team at our research centre in Newcastle burst excitedly into my office, clutching a pair of images. Dr Mavin Macauley had spent two years measuring the size of the pancreas in people with type 2 diabetes. It had been a struggle. But now he had started to measure the pancreas in people without diabetes. And he could not believe his eyes.

There it was, obvious at a glance. All the pancreases Mavin had come across so far in people with type 2 diabetes were small and ragged. We had both assumed that this was what the pancreas always looked like. But here, in people without diabetes, were two lovely plump, smooth pancreases. Eureka!

Moments like these are rare in science, and to be enjoyed. Medical research is 99% perspiration and 1% inspiration, with the occasional episode of huge excitement. The picture below shows pancreases from two similar people, one of whom has type 2 diabetes. You can see just what Mavin was so excited about. It does not take an expert to spot the difference.

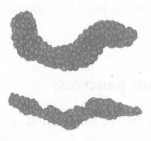

Even now, very few diabetes specialists know that a person with type 2 diabetes has a shrunken pancreas. It is only just beginning to be talked about, and comes as a surprise to many doctors.

Why is the pancreas smaller in type 2 diabetes? Looking at those images that day, we thought there were two possibilities. On the one hand, it was possible that people who had been born with rather small pancreases were more prone to type 2 diabetes. On the other hand, perhaps the same thing had caused the pancreas to shrink and caused the diabetes itself? We had to find out. And we did! We now know that the pancreas shrinks as diabetes develops. But crucially, and very excitingly, we also know that it can grow back to normal size slowly over about two years once a person loses weight and returns to normal blood sugar control.

In this chapter I've explained how the body works in normal life, before diabetes comes on. In the next section I will explain what happens when the pancreas cannot do its job any more – and why.

Quick read

- Food is essential for life, but can be poisonous if too much is eaten over a long period of time

- Just a little too much food over many years causes fat to build up inside the liver and pancreas

- When the liver is too fatty, it pumps out too much sugar and too much fat to the rest of the body

- Fat then builds up inside the pancreas, and it cannot make enough insulin at the right time

- Result: too much sugar in the blood

- The pancreas is the most important organ in diabetes

Chapter 4

Your Personal Fat Threshold

Only one in two of all people with type 2 diabetes is actually obese. And if we test even very overweight people, 3 out of 4 do not have the disease.

Let's have a reality check.

Why me? Why have I got type 2 diabetes?

Rene Laennec was the famous French doctor who invented the stethoscope. He used to say to his students: 'Listen to your patients. They are giving you the diagnosis.' But he was not talking about listening to the heart or lungs. He was talking about the most important skill of a doctor – listening. Listening to the story a patient tells about what has happened and what has caused them to seek medical advice. This story, to the expert ear, leads to an understanding of the sort of disease that has caused a patient's symptoms. This is the basis of being a good doctor. It is a message still relevant today.

When the results of my first study on reversing type 2 diabetes were reported in the media in 2011, I received a huge number of emails from people with diabetes telling me about their condition, how long they had had it, what complications they had experienced and whether it was well controlled. Many people just wanted to learn how they could get rid of their diabetes. But there were lots who emailed to say that they were not overweight but had still developed the disease. It was something I had heard frequently in my clinic: 'Why have I got type 2 diabetes when my friends are all fatter than me and they don't?'

It is indeed confusing: it is known that people who do not look too heavy can get type 2 diabetes. And yet at the same time we know that type 2 diabetes is directly caused by excess fat in the body. So what is going on?

Let me tell you about Mark, a patient of mine from whom I learned a lot. I met Mark early on, when I was just beginning to understand what caused type 2 diabetes. He was outraged that diabetes had happened to him; he was not obese, not even overweight. He had come to me to see if there was any way of getting rid of it. By this time, I already knew that people with type 2 diabetes had fatty livers. We performed some blood tests, which showed that Mark's liver was not as healthy as it should have been, probably because it contained too much fat – even though he didn't look fat overall. And it was at this point that I figured out that it was specifically the high levels of *liver* fat that might be the main problem, rather than how much fat was on show on the outside. If this was true, it could point a way forwards for Mark. Even though he looked as if he was of normal weight, why not suggest major weight loss as a possible way of getting rid of his liver fat to see if this improved the control of his sugar levels?

I gave this unusual advice to Mark, warning him that there were no guarantees of success, but explaining that it was the only possible way I could think of to help him achieve his aim: to get rid of his diabetes. Over 2,000 years ago, Hippocrates laid down the vital principle for doctors: 'At least do no harm.' Losing weight would do no harm to Mark, and he was desperate to try to get back to normal. He agreed to do it.

So 'normal-weight' Mark lost weight. His BMI went down from 24 to just below 20. And the diabetes went away.

It went away!

As I had expected, his blood sugar first thing in the morning returned to normal due to the reduction in liver fat. However, I was surprised to see that his blood sugar levels after meals also went back to normal. This set my brain buzzing. It could only mean that the pancreas had improved, too. Wow! Was it possible that the pancreas as well as the liver had been gummed up with fat? If so, I was looking at the very cause of type 2 diabetes.

So, fast forward to 2011, when the dramatic results of our first study on the cause of type 2 diabetes hit the newspapers and all those emails came in. The most heartfelt ones (and some angry ones) were from people with type 2 diabetes who had a 'normal' BMI. Because of my research results and the good effect on Mark, it seemed reasonable to reply that losing weight might reverse their type 2 diabetes too.

By email, a doctor can only give information – not personal medical advice – and it is essential not to get in the way of someone's own doctor. So we limited ourselves to providing the information we had about the effect of losing weight, and everyone was advised to discuss the way forward with their own doctor or nurse.

You may guess what happened next. In a couple of months emails arrived from these 'normal-weight' people saying that after losing weight their sugar levels had returned to normal too. Many testified that they had made an appointment with their doctor or nurse to discuss the weight loss plan in advance, as advised, and been told, 'Don't do it! It would be unhealthy to lose weight as your BMI is already in the normal range.' But the desire to escape from type 2 diabetes was so strong that they ignored this well-meaning advice. One of them was a journalist, and he wrote about his experience. His article helped a considerable number of people.

Why 'normal-weight' people may be too heavy for their own body

The word 'normal' crops up a lot when describing people. But in my scientific life, I have found that fixed limits can often be too restrictive. There really is no one size which fits all. Perhaps we need to shake off this politically correct idea that a certain level of anything is normal and that to be above or below that is bad. A 'normal' BMI is defined as less than 25. But just look at your fellow human beings in the street. Some look like rugby players, and some like they might be long-distance runners. We come in all shapes and sizes.

What, I reasoned, if those who did not look chubby on the outside actually had too much fat on the inside? This notion had previously been described as TOFI – Thin Outside, Fat Inside. But now, thanks to Mark, the people who emailed and my research, I knew we were on to something big: that people with type 2 diabetes who did not look too heavy had nonetheless very probably been much thinner when they were 20–25 years old, and their weight gain was effectively 'invisible'.

Did Mark become abnormally thin after losing weight in his bid to rid himself of his type 2? Not at all – or at least not for him. In fact, his weight had merely returned to what it was in his early twenties. In the two decades since then, he had gradually accumulated more fat than he could safely store, and he had become unable to cope with the amount of fat in his liver and pancreas. His weight had become too high *for him* – even though it was unremarkable compared with what was 'normal' for most other people.

The whole episode set me thinking about the so-called 'normal' range for the whole population. What if each person had an individual level of tolerance for levels of fat in the body, with problems starting if this level was exceeded? I called this the Personal Fat Threshold concept. PFT for short.

Just look at the population

In the 1970s and '80s, the population of the UK was considerably lighter than at present. In fact, accurate surveys have shown that, between 1980 and 2012, the average weight of both men and women increased by about one and a half stone (9.5kg) – a huge change. In

1980, the general population had an average BMI of 24. Can you remember what people looked like then? Have a look at the picture below.

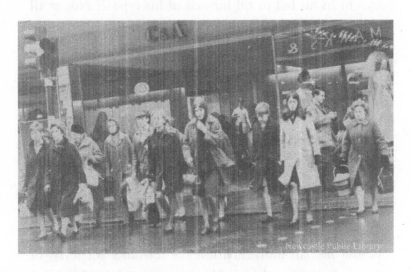

People on the street in Newcastle in the late 1970s. It was rare to see an overweight person. Reproduced with permission from Newcastle Public Library.

Let's look at what has happened in only 32 years. In 1980, according to a survey of the adult population of England and Wales, only one in every 14 people (7%) had a BMI over 30 and would be labelled obese. In 2012, this careful survey was repeated. By then the proportion of the population with a BMI over 30 had shot up to one in four people, or by 25%. These statistics sound shocking: a huge increase in obesity rates in just three decades! What was wrong with these people? it was asked. Well, nothing actually. The increase in weight was not restricted to those who became obese. Almost *everyone* has become heavier. Look at this:

- People who used to have a BMI of 35 now have a BMI of 38. They are more obese.
- People who used to have a BMI of 29 now have a BMI of 31. They have become 'obese'.
- Those who used to have a BMI of 24 now have a BMI of 27. They have become 'overweight'.
- Slightly built people have increased their BMI from 19 to 22. They are still labelled 'normal'.

This summary is useful, but it is only talking about averages. Of course, some people have gained more than others. How keen is your appetite? How ravenous do you get? Your 'appetite' reflects your luck of the draw in terms of which genes you inherited. People born with the most active appetites are superbly suited for survival during food scarcity – though tend to put on the most weight when food is available. But we need to see the difference between individuals and the population as a whole. Within any population, an individual is heavier or lighter than others mainly because of their genes. But when we look at whole populations, it is a question of how readily food is available – ie the environment they live in – that determines the 'average' weight.

The reality is that the environment in which we live has changed, and the population is changing as a result. This was neatly captured in a few words in a Lancet article in 2002: 'The obesity epidemic is due to normal people doing normal things in an abnormal environment.'

There are some who claim that everyone has personal responsibility for their own health, that anyone letting their weight get too high is just irresponsible. But in reality, thinking about future health is not the number one concern day-to-day for most people. Those who are well off can devote much time and thought every day to keeping weight down, eating carefully or taking exercise. But for the majority of folk life intervenes: things like illness in the family, money worries, family problems, work demands, a leaking roof, friends in trouble. These all crowd in – and what, when and how much we eat is not at the forefront of our minds every moment of the day.

In our modern world, the constant availability of food, and being surrounded by others eating at any time, at home, at work and even in the street, makes it all too easy to eat mindlessly. Like it or not, most of our lives run on autopilot, and it is difficult to battle against what everyone else seems to be doing.

The PFT – it is about YOU not the 'average'

It is all very well talking about the average weight gain of the entire population. But we are all individuals, and your doctor has only one person – just you – sitting in front of them in a consultation. What matters is *your* PFT.

Let's just imagine some of the individuals in the population. The picture below shows some people arranged according to their BMI. Some people are skinny, some are a bit chunkier and some are large. Not everyone can be a champion jockey – those slim-build individuals are all on the left-hand side of the line-up. Equally, not everyone can be a rugby player or weight lifter – they are more over on the right. There is a wide range of normal.

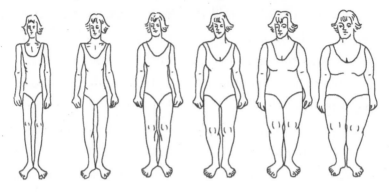

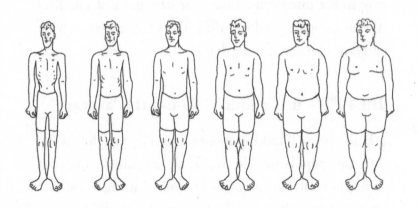

Now let's meet three men who have developed type 2 diabetes:

Jack is heavy. His doctor told him that his BMI is 38.

Joe thought his weight was normal and was told his BMI is 29.

Harry looks slim and was told his BMI is 24.

According to the officially fixed cut-offs for BMI, Jack would be told he was obese. Bad boy – must lose weight. Joe would be told that he is overweight but not obese; maybe shed a pound or two. Harry would be told that he was normal and that he should not lose weight.

But hang on a minute! We need to consider what had happened over the 20 years or so before their diabetes was diagnosed. This is shown in the picture below. Like most people in their forties, each had put on weight since they were younger. Jack at the age of 21 did not look like Harry at the same age! They all started from different weights, and each of them had increased their BMI by about three units.

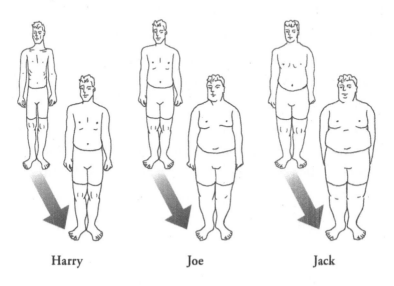

Harry   Joe   Jack

We now know that each of these men had crossed their PFT. They had all become too heavy for their own bodies. Through no fault of his own, Harry was more susceptible to just a moderate amount of fat. Joe was a bit less susceptible and Jack would have been fine – but pushed it too far.

I've changed their names, but these three men are all real people whom I have advised. They all lost weight and they all reversed their diabetes. Jack lost almost two and a half stone (15kg) and reduced his BMI from 38 to 35.

Joe lost the same (two and a half stone/15kg) and shifted his BMI from 29 to 26. And Harry, who started with a BMI of 24, lost just under two stone (12kg) to get down to a BMI of 21.

If we asked a statistics expert what had happened, they would say, 'Nothing. Just look at the numbers. Jack is still obese (BMI over 30). Joe is still overweight (BMI 25–30). Harry is still normal weight.' You can see how fixed cut-offs that put people into boxes can be misleading. The lesson is, if you want advice about your own health, do not consult a statistician! They do a great job of describing populations – but you are you.

So what does the PFT really mean? It means that we all have our own tolerance for weight gain. Some people have positively athletic fat tissue under the skin – which can handle anything thrown at it, with apparently endless storage capacity. Lucky people, we might say. They are Nature's survivors who will do well during any famine or other disaster. Of course, as they acquire more and more fat it may look excessive, but it is stored away safely. The trouble controlling blood sugar starts when fat can no longer be stored safely and spills over into the liver and then the pancreas. And that is not safe.

A big study of nurses in the United States backs up my story about Jack, Joe and Harry. It showed that, while those who had stayed close to the weight they were in their early twenties remained free of type 2 diabetes, those who put on weight, even within the 'normal' BMI range, were four times more likely to develop type 2 diabetes.

So let's forget all talk of type 2 diabetes as a disease of 'obesity'. The fact is that, at the time of diagnosis of type 2 diabetes, one in ten people have a 'normal' BMI (under 25). I should point out that these numbers are for people of white European ethnicity. Typical body shapes are different in people of South Asian or Far Eastern ethnicity, and the number of people in these communities getting type 2 diabetes is much higher at a BMI level that is lower than usually regarded as 'normal' (ie 25). In other words, the PFT is usually lower in these ethnic groups. Both the NHS and the American Diabetes Association recommend different BMI levels for people of South Asian or Far Eastern ethnicity:

- 'Normal'   18.5 to 23
- Overweight   23 to 27.5
- Obese   over 27.5

The exact reason for the differences between different ethnicities is not fully understood, but knowing they exist can be very helpful. Incidentally, just as people of white ethnicity, like my former patient Mark, can develop type

2 when they have what is regarded as a normal BMI of 25, people of South Asian or Far Eastern ethnicity can develop type 2 diabetes at a BMI officially described as 'normal' for them, i.e. 19. Surely you can't get type 2 diabetes with a BMI of 19? Yes you can! The bottom line is the same for everyone: type 2 diabetes develops when your PFT is exceeded.

Another point to note: whatever your ethnicity, it can be very useful to measure around your waist as this is often a better guide to a risk of diabetes. Men are at risk of type 2 diabetes if their waist circumference is more than 35 inches (89cm), and women are at risk if over 31.5 inches (80cm).

Too heavy for your body

Samuel Johnson had a neat way with words and was a keen observer of people. Around 1790 he said, 'If a man is too fat, it is plain for all to see that he has eaten more than he should have done.'

He did not say that the person had 'eaten too much'. He recognised that different people required different amounts of food, and that some people could become too heavy *for their own body*. Johnson's words provide a neat summing up of the cause of type 2 diabetes.

Quick read

- Type 2 diabetes is not caused by 'obesity'

- Everyone has a Personal Fat Threshold of weight above which they might develop type 2 diabetes

- This is determined mainly by the genes controlling how much fat you can store safely under the skin

- Above that limit, excess fat will spill over to the liver, then to the pancreas

- The stop/go for type 2 diabetes is inside your beta cells, which may or may not be susceptible to the bad effects of excess fat

- Even if you are unlucky and have both a low storage space for fat *and* fat-susceptible beta cells, remember: no excess fat, no diabetes

Part III

HOW TO ESCAPE FROM TYPE 2 DIABETES

Chapter 5

Planning your escape

In the next chapter, I am going to outline the 1–2–3 diet, originally devised for volunteers in our research studies on diabetes reversal. It was so successful that it is now used by doctors for treatment of the disease. This is a three-step programme involving: first, rapid weight loss, where you eat a combination of low-calorie soups or shakes with some salad or leafy vegetables, adding up to 700–800 calories daily for a period of eight weeks; second, a gradual reintroduction of normal meals; and third, a return to a pattern of normal eating, one which is sustainable in the long term.

Before we get on to the nitty gritty of the diet itself, though, we need to prepare for what's ahead. Losing a lot of weight quickly is highly motivating, but it can be a challenge, so you need to make a firm decision about whether or not you really want to do it, and plan in advance for how you will manage to stay on course.

1. Recognise the problem

For centuries, type 2 diabetes was thought of as a life-long condition. Big studies showed an inevitable downhill path, regardless of what tablets were given. We now know that it can be reversed. So why did earlier studies on the disease 'prove' that type 2 diabetes always progressed and never went away? The simple answer is that people did not lose weight. In fact, the opposite usually happened. Because in real life, even though they are usually advised to lose some weight, people with type 2 diabetes find that their weight just continues to creep up.

This may not surprise you if you have been on the receiving end of routine advice about weight loss. It is often handed out with no conviction that it will work, or given without a clear explanation as to how to follow it. Certainly, doctors are not surprised that most people's weight steadily increases after being diagnosed with type 2, because they know that some of the tablets used for diabetes actually cause them to put weight on.

As we have seen, tablets can improve blood glucose levels for a while, but they do not stop the progression of the disease, because the insulin-producing cells inside the pancreas are slowly being poisoned by accumulated fat. How much fat? Half a gram. That small amount of excess fat is inside the cells, preventing the proper manufacture and release of insulin. At the same time, there is too much fat in the blood, which is continuously arriving and adding to the burden.

Now, you might think that there must be some clever way of targeting this small amount of fat that is in the wrong place. Sadly, there is not. The only way of getting rid of this fat is to decrease the total amount of fat in your body – not just by a few pounds, but by a lot. Once you have understood this, escape from type 2 diabetes is within your grasp. You must lose a significant amount of weight and then keep it off.

2. Write down how much weight you need to lose

However much fat you have in your body, the development of type 2 diabetes is telling you that you have too much. Too much for *you*. Don't compare your size with that of others. You are yourself. Your 'constitution' is different from other people's, you have a different Personal Fat Threshold.

As a rule of thumb, decreasing your body weight by two and a half stone (about 15kg) will be sufficient to take you below your PFT. That is for most people. If you are not a big person it may be too much. You can still be above your PFT yet not heavy, compared with others. If you weigh less than 12 and a half stone, it is better to think about losing a certain percentage of your body weight (about 10%). Have a look at the table below. Someone weighing ten stone (63kg) might more reasonably aim to lose about one and a half stone (9.5kg).

Either way, to strip the internal fat from your organs and reverse type 2 diabetes, you need to lose a significant amount of weight. As you read this, right now, this may sound an impossible task. But I can assure you it is easier than you may think. The people who helped in our research found that cutting their calorie intake to 700–800 calories daily was far easier than they had expected. It surprised me too! Compared with the miserable and often ineffective business of trying to lose weight over six months or a year, losing a lot of weight rapidly was found to be genuinely more acceptable. What helps is the speed of your early weight loss: you lose around half a stone (3.2kg) in the first week. This makes a huge difference to how you feel day to day. Just try to get up out of a chair, or walk upstairs while carrying a bag weighing half a stone. Then do the same without. All daily activities become very suddenly much easier when you are lighter. Stairs? What stairs? You will feel so much better so quickly that your motivation will be reinforced.

Yes, you will feel very hungry for the first 36 hours, but hardly at all after that. That is one of the biggest surprises for people who have followed this plan. The main problems are about adjusting daily life around the major changes you will have to make while you in the first phase of the diet:

- you can't join in with family mealtimes or other social eating
- you should avoid eating with others at work
- you need to ensure that when you are out of the house you are prepared and will not end up buying something on the hoof.

For most people, it is the same whether you weigh 12 stone or 24 stone. Losing two and a half stone is highly likely to return your sugar control to normal. It is true that some people have had their type 2 diabetes for too long and may not be able to reverse it, but this applies to only 10% of people who are still within the first six years of diagnosis. The only way to find out whether your diabetes has gone too far to be reversed is to lose the weight and see. I know two people who had type 2 diabetes for 23 years but successfully escaped.

The aim is not to become slim (although for some this may be a happy by-product!). What is important is to get rid of your diabetes – to get yourself below your PFT. Of course, there may be other health gains to be had from losing even more weight, but this book is about getting rid of diabetes, not becoming a fashion model.

The first step is to find your current weight on the table, and then read off what your weight needs to be. This is your target weight. Write it down. Then it is a real target.

As I say, don't be put off by the seemingly impossible job – hundreds of people like you have achieved this amount of weight loss. It can be done. Just like moving to the long-term home of your dreams, you should start looking forward to it.

Your weight now:		What it needs to be:	
Stones/pounds	Kilos	Stones/pounds	Kilos
23 8	150	21 3	135
22 11	145	20 6	130
22 0	140	19 9	125
21 3	135	18 12	120
20 6	130	18 1	115
19 9	125	17 4	110
18 12	120	16 7	105
18 1	115	15 10	100

Your weight now:			What it needs to be:		
Stones/pounds		Kilos	Stones/pounds		Kilos
17	4	110	14	13	95
16	7	105	14	2	90
15	10	100	13	5	85
14	13	95	12	8	80
14	2	90	11	11	75
13	5	85	11	0	70
12	8	80	10	6	65
11	11	75	10	0	64
11	0	70	9	4	60
10	3	65	8	9	55
9	6	60	8	0	51

3. Recognise that you must eat less for two months

When will you start on your escape diet? Certainly not right now. You need to plan ahead. This is not an invitation to put the start date off, then postpone it again, but rather to encourage you to take a cool look ahead to check that you are making things as easy as possible for yourself. Choose your time. You may struggle to find two months when there are no social occasions, upheavals at work, holidays etc. Perhaps you have a family party in a few weeks' time? In which case, earmark the least difficult time, and, if you do have an event to factor in, there are a number of things you can do to prevent it blowing you off course.

- Take your own food or shake
- Make sure to drink only water or zero calorie beverages
- Leave before the food is served

Some of our volunteers told me that they would have their liquid meal to ensure they felt full before going out to an event. Then they wouldn't let a morsel pass their lips during the do. Enlisting support from everyone close to you will be extremely helpful.

If you want to take part in a more extended event – say, a special weekend – that might prove extra challenging, there is always the option of taking a break from your diet. But remember that this is the more difficult way: that brief diet 'holiday' will be followed by a further 36 hours of feeling hungry again as your body re-acclimatises. From everything that our research volunteers have told us, breaks from the diet should be the exception. They should be reserved for only very, very special occasions. Otherwise, there is a risk that the diet 'holidays' start to feel acceptable and habitual eating creeps back in and hampers your escape effort.

The decision regarding how to make this work has to be yours. But do remember that learning how to manage social occasions involving food and drink is a valuable skill for the future. Indeed it will stand you in good stead for ever.

4. Talk to friends and family

It is really important to get the support of family and friends before you embark on this programme, since planning major weight loss affects them too. Eating is a social activity, and usually involves your nearest and dearest. Many families eat together as a routine. What did you do last time you met a friend? You probably had a drink or something to eat with them, just as a normal part of the occasion. So be aware that any change you make to what and how much you eat will impinge upon everyone else in your life.

You should find family, friends and colleagues are supportive: how could they not be happy to see you not only reversing your diabetes but ending up considerably lighter and feeling ten years younger? Well, it does happen. Sometimes a spouse/partner/close friend may feel ambivalent about you embarking on this challenge. Or even positively against it. They might feel that there is a message in it for them – perhaps because they are a good deal heavier than they were 20 years ago and do not want to face the fact that the extra weight is not doing them any good.

In our early studies only three people dropped out, and in all cases the reason was that their spouse/partner did not want them to lose more weight. This may surprise you, but remember that those close to you may prefer you as you are. After all, it is reassuring when people around us do not change. So you need to be prepared for this too, and try and bring them on board.

A family decision to avoid eating anything other than at meal times is a good first step. In today's overfed society snacking between meals has become the norm; we are tempted at every turn by biscuits and cakes and sugary hot drinks. But just 50 years ago this sort of overfeeding would have seemed absurd. Can you tell the difference between boredom and real hunger? Often if you say, 'I feel a bit peckish', it really means 'nothing much doing just now'. Learn to spot the difference.

Temptation is much easier to deal with if you remove it. We often hear people talk about the bad environment we live in – meaning our use of cars, our labour-saving machines and our ready access to fast foods. But it is easy to overlook the bad micro-environment of our own homes. That environment can be changed if the family is willing. Many of our research volunteers have described this revolution.

Beware such excuses as 'I need to keep some treats in the cupboards for the children/grandchildren!' Beware these excuses. Remember, firstly, that type 2 diabetes runs in families, and your youngsters will share your genes. They are at risk of developing type 2 diabetes in later life. So having 'treats' as a routine will do them no favours in the long term. It would be far better to actively help them avoid having to make the same escape effort that you are thinking about just now.

Secondly, if you are tempted to eat the treats, then they were probably never really for the kids anyway. Be honest: if you are unable to resist them, they will have to go.

5. Decide whether to do it

How do you make a decision? Some people weigh up all the facts, ponder on them for a while and carefully come to a conclusion. Other people – probably most – come to a snap decision either immediately on hearing the pros and cons or later triggered by some other factor.

Consider how you would reach a decision about a different health issue. Imagine if, instead of diabetes, you had developed a life-threatening disease which could only be cured by an operation and your doctor said to you,

'If you want to stay alive, you have to take three months off work to recover from the operation and stop all your normal activities.' Faced with a life-threatening condition, you would not hesitate to accept this. It would be a no-brainer. You would plan for the operation and work out how to fit your life around this period of down time.

In view of all the misery and shortening of life caused by diabetes that I described in Chapter 1, doesn't it make sense to weigh up the pros and cons just as you would if you were facing a life-saving operation? Diabetes threatens your eyesight, your feet and your heart, not to mention doubling the risk of a stroke at any age. And there are other bad things about diabetes. You have acquired a disease label. Unthinkingly, people now say that you are 'a diabetic'. You will end up spending ages in your doctor's waiting room. Your holiday insurance will cost twice as much. You face a lifetime of monitoring and medication.

And when you think about it, the way to fix diabetes is much less disruptive than, say, three months off work for an operation. During your period of low-calorie dieting, work and everyday life will continue. You may worry that you won't have enough energy to do your usual work, but do not fear – most people report feeling *more* energetic than usual while dieting. Our research volunteers said they felt much livelier than before. Yes, a few did experience some tiredness (about one in 15), but they were still able to continue working, even doing physically demanding jobs. The potential prize at the end kept them motivated and made their efforts feel worthwhile.

I could come up with any number of reasons to try to persuade you that following this programme is a good idea. But it is a challenge; and ultimately it is you who has to reach that decision. Some people may feel that they would prefer just to take the pills and accept whatever fate has in store for them. Fair enough. It is not obligatory to try and reverse your condition, and may not be practical for some people. It has to be a personal choice. But in my experience most people would really like to have their health back – as soon as possible. Health is one of those things that we do not value until we lose it.

Don't forget the previous point about enlisting the support of family and friends. Do talk it over with your spouse, partner and work colleagues. Ideally, everyone will get behind your mission, if not actively involved.

But whatever the process for you, and however wide-ranging the discussion, a decision needs to be taken. Don't rush through this step. You will know when you have decided. And provided you have been given the information about the alternatives, no one can tell you that your decision is 'wrong' or 'right'. Just be sure that you are sure.

6. Prepare for action

Check those cupboards. Are they clear of biscuits, cakes and crisps? Do you have all the supplies you need? Packets to make up liquid meals? Salad stuff and other non-starchy veg? Bottles of fizzy water in the fridge? If you work away from home, it would be a good idea to stock up on packed lunch equipment – Tupperware for salads, thermal mugs for soup – so you can be forearmed. It is essential to plan ahead so you don't get scuppered by circumstances and end up buying a calorie-heavy snack.

Likewise, be ready to deal with any ambushing. If you have a friend, relative or acquaintance who seems to want to sabotage your efforts to lose weight – 'You will have a muffin, won't you?' 'I'm dying for a pint, aren't you?' – you need to have a plan for how you will respond. It can be a particularly difficult thing to deal with when you are doing your best to keep to a strict regime. Certainly, I could hardly believe it when my patients first described this problem to me; but it is real and it happens.

7. Action!

All our work on reversing type 2 diabetes at Newcastle University has depended upon finding a method for losing weight that can be achieved by everyone within a short period of time. To make a research study work, the method chosen has to be acceptable to most people. And we found that eight weeks on a combination of low-calorie complete nutrition shakes plus a portion of non-starchy vegetables adding up to 700–800 calories worked really well. But you are not 'most people'. You are an individual and, for a range of reasons, you may be able to achieve the vital goal – two and a half stone weight loss – by other means. Perhaps you hate the idea of low-calorie drinks, and would rather cook for yourself. That is fine. Whatever works for you.

The key thing is that you need to mentally prepare yourself not just for the period of intense dieting but also for long-term weight control – right from the beginning. You must be prepared for the fact that, once you have shed that two and a half stone and after you have congratulated yourself (and your supporters), you will need to eat less food than you previously ate. In practice, this will be around three-quarters of the amount you used to put on your plate by habit. And you will need to do this for ever.

Remember, this marks the beginning of the rest of your life. And eating less will be the only way to maintain your new, healthy, slimmer form.

Quick read

- 1. Recognise the problem:
  If you have type 2 diabetes you have become too heavy for your body

- 2. Write down your target weight:
  Usually a weight loss of 15kg or two and a half stone

- 3. Recognise that food intake has to be decreased for 2-3 months:
  Think when it may suit you to do this

- 4. Discuss with family and friends:
  Support is one of the secrets of success

- 5. Decide:
  Do you really want to do this?

- 6. Prepare for action:
  Clear the cupboards

- 7. Action:
  Do it.

Chapter 6

The 1–2–3 approach

Now that you understand why diabetes occurs and that it is possible to return to full health, I am going to outline the 3-step approach we developed for diabetes reversal at Newcastle University. It really is as simple as 1, 2, 3:

1. Lose weight rapidly on a low-calorie regime over two months, focusing entirely on that
2. Reintroduce ordinary foods gradually over a month
3. Keep the weight down long term.

Losing a significant amount of weight in a short time followed by keeping weight steady is very different from the standard advice. What has been advised for years is to cut back a *little* on what you eat and to lose weight gradually. In practice, this leaves you hungry for ever. It is prolonged torture for many. And it clearly does not work for most people.

In contrast, the 1–2–3 approach recognises that losing weight is a distinct activity. One that is separate from the long-term matter of keeping your weight steady. Careful research has shown that it is much easier to lose a large amount of weight rapidly than you would expect, and there are many benefits. Hunger is not usually a big problem with this plan. You will start feeling good after only a week or two. That reinforces your determination to succeed. During the course of the eight weeks you can expect to lose about two and a half stone (15kg).

In the early studies looking into what caused type 2 diabetes, I had to come up with a sure-fire way to get our volunteers to lose a lot of weight. I devised a programme of eight weeks on low-calorie powdered shakes together with some non-starchy vegetables (see the list below), which provided all the necessary protein, minerals and micronutrients in a daily quota of 700-800 calories. However, after our first trial, our research volunteers told us of the difficulty they had had in re-starting normal eating after this rapid weight loss phase. They described how, after eight weeks of simply choosing which shake flavour to make up in water, they did not know what to do and felt panicky when trying to prepare a meal. So for our next trial we added a clearly laid out, second step to the programme, whereby over the course of a month you replace each of your three daily shakes with a meal of ordinary food. From then on the 3-step programme looked like this:

Step 1 - Rapid weight loss - 8 weeks.
Consumption to be limited to 700-800 calories daily. The simplest option is to use a liquid formula product providing around 600 calories per day, plus a plateful of non-starchy vegetables - 100-200 calories approximately (see box below). No alcohol - and no change to exercise.

Step 2 - Return to normal eating - 4 weeks
For two weeks, one small meal of ordinary foods (of 400-500 calories) is substituted for the evening liquid meal. For the second two weeks, you do the same for lunch (with a meal of around 400 calories). At the four-week mark, breakfast is reintroduced and all shakes are stopped.

Step 3. Long-term weight maintenance
Eating is back to being a normal, social activity - but with a close eye on quantities. The same goes for alcohol. From now on you should be consuming about three quarters of what you used to eat. Your weighing scales are your best friend.

We used this approach, which became known as the 'Newcastle diet', in our next research study and were pleased to find that all our volunteers found it much easier. Added to which, their weight stayed steady during the six months of follow-up. It ought to be said here that Step 3 is the most challenging – if you want to keep type 2 diabetes at bay, weight regain has to be avoided for life.

Food v liquid formula

Replacing a meal with a complete nutrition drink from a packet is by far the easiest option for most people. There are lots of brands available in supermarkets and chemists. Most have a wide range of flavours to choose from and minimise boredom. As part of the 'Newcastle diet', we advised everyone to add in some non-starchy vegetables, partly for something to chew on (people like doing this!) but mainly because veg helps to prevent constipation.

There are other ways of going about the low-calorie weight loss phase, though. If you want, you could miss out the vegetables but add in a fourth packet of liquid formula. This may be simpler. But constipation is likely so you will have to take regular laxatives.

And, if you can't bear the idea of going on

liquid formula drinks for several weeks with or without vegetables, you can of course use ordinary foods. You would have to make up meals containing around 200 calories, with no more than 800 calories a day. This involves a lot of planning and preparation time in the kitchen, and many people find it more difficult because of the daily burden of decisions and choices.

If you go for real foods giving you 800 calories per day, you will need to include a lot of protein foods (fish, meat, cheese). This is important not only to ensure that you meet your daily need for protein (about 50g for an adult), but also because these foods keep you more satisfied for longer. As do non-starchy vegetables which give a feeling of plenty because of their high-fibre content. It may take you a bit longer to cruise down to your target weight – about three to four months instead of two months on the liquid formula. There is also a possibility on any food-based diet of 800 calories per day that you could run short on some vitamins, and for this reason you should take a multivitamin tablet.

There are whole books devoted entirely to low-calorie eating, and such approaches can suit some people very well. This is not rocket science. If you can achieve rapid weight loss simply by a drastic reduction in the amount of food that you eat at every meal, then that is fine.

What are non-starchy vegetables?

Artichoke	Fennel	Samphire
Asparagus	Gherkins	Sugar snap peas
Aubergine	Green beans	Sauerkraut
Beansprouts	Leeks	Shallots
Broad beans	Lettuce	Spinach
Broccoli	Mange tout	Spring greens
Brussels sprouts	Marrow	Spring onions
Cabbage	Mushrooms	Squash
Carrots	Okra	Swede
Cauliflower	Onions	Tomatoes (fresh
Cavolo Nero	Pak choi	or tinned)
Celeriac	Pea shoots	Turnips
Celery	Peppers	Watercress
Courgette	Radishes	
Cucumber	Rocket	

Any spices or herbs can be added to make the flavour of your veg or salad more interesting. Very small amounts (1 teaspoonful) of olive oil or mayonnaise can also be added – once per day.

How to do it – Step 1

Choose your low-calorie diet. If it is to be a liquid diet, then you must decide which brand you are going to use and which flavours you like. Whichever you choose it must say that it provides 'complete nutrition' – in other words, all the vitamins, minerals and trace elements in addition to protein, sugar and fat. You may be surprised by the high sugar content of some brands – but don't worry as this is tiny compared with what your liver makes every day. The protein content will be high – around 25% – much higher than usually eaten. It must come as one packet per meal (no decisions or room for inadvertently adjusted doses).

As I say, a liquid diet is easier for most people, and bear in mind that this is what was used in our research which showed major weight loss and lasting remission of type 2 diabetes. I steer clear of recommending any particular brands because it is important for me as a doctor and scientist to be entirely unbiased. But I am often asked for examples of suitable products.

Exante, and Optifast are made up with water. The Kee Diet and Superdrug Slender Plan need to be made up with semi-skimmed milk. The prices vary so do shop around and find a brand that suits your taste.

If you are going for the ordinary food option, or even a mixture of the two, you will need to be well prepared, with the right ingredients and recipes to keep you going. And be realistic: you will not want to spend hours preparing gourmet low-calories meals every day. So have some quick, easy, calorie-counted options at the ready

– you can't go wrong with some grilled chicken or fish and a pile of non-starchy vegetables, for example. Make this your default main meal every day if need be.

Other tips to help you manage this step:

- Write down why you are doing this. This can be useful to read later when you may be struggling to keep up with the demands of daily life while also avoiding putting weight back on.

- During a liquid diet, you will have lots of time on your hands as you won't be preparing food and perhaps won't even be sitting at the family table at meal times, so think in advance about what you are going to do with that time.

- Do not suddenly start a new exercise programme when you are on Step 1. Perhaps surprisingly, this can seriously impede weight loss, especially in very overweight people. This is probably the best-kept secret in the weight loss field, and I only found out about it by listening to people helping with one of our exercise studies. Bouts of hard exercise make you feel hungry and tend to induce 'compensatory eating' (part conscious and part subconscious). So just carry on doing whatever activity you normally do during Step 1 - don't try to do more.

- What are you going to do if you do feel tempted to eat something off-limits? Writing a list of distractions can be helpful - jobs around the house, surprising the dog with an extra walk, drinking a pint of water, planning future holidays.

- You also need to plan for how to supply yourself with your special meals when out of the house. This is easiest if your chosen liquid diet powder is designed to be dissolved in water rather than milk, but advance planning will make things more manageable in either case.

- No alcohol during the weight loss phase. Alcohol is high in calories. Think of it as liquid fat. Not helpful. Just don't do it.

- Continue to enjoy tea and coffee, with skimmed milk (not more than 1.7fl oz per day) if preferred.

- Do discuss your plans with your doctor or diabetes nurse.

What people say about Step 1

These are some of the things people said about their experience of the liquid diet in our early studies:

'I was so surprised. When I compare what I have been eating over the last weeks to what I used to eat I really would have thought that I would have been hungry from the moment I opened my eyes to the moment I closed my eyes, but I wasn't.' (Woman, aged 42 years, one year after reversing to normal).

'It was fairly hard to start with, but it got easier as the weeks went on and when I started getting a bit fitter and I could walk further and stand up and sit down and dig the garden it was great. I feel great.' (Man, aged 44 years, two and a half years since diagnosis).

Although the majority reflected these thoughts, not everyone found it feasible:

'I was in town at one point, bakeries everywhere, smells of people eating all around you and, it was ridiculous, I couldn't concentrate. I would have been fine if I had been at home, I would have lost weight this week and still been on it, but I couldn't stick to it.' (Man, aged 52 years, one year since diagnosis).

The next quote reflects what has happened to our high streets over the last two to three decades. This person was not alone in lamenting the all-pervasive offerings of food in our environment today:

'You just can't get away from food. Pick up the paper and there is Jamie Oliver doing something clever with a leg of lamb. So turn on the telly, and there is Mary Berry baking cakes. So you take yourself off to the football, only to find yourself surrounded by hamburger adverts and stalls. I couldn't sit at the family dinner table. I had to fill in time by going to the cinema to watch just anything. Poor sad old geezer sitting by himself. But it worked.' (Man, aged 57 years, still free of diabetes three years after finishing the study).

How to do it – Step 2

Just as there is a clear focus during the initial weight loss phase, there is a definite plan for the month-long food re-introduction phase, whereby first you replace your evening shake with a small meal, then after two weeks of this you introduce another small meal to replace your lunchtime shake, and then finally add in breakfast and stop all the shakes.

A few things to note while you are on this phase:

- Your start-up dinner should be around half the amount you would have previously eaten - around 400-500 calories. For instance, it might be a normal amount of meat or fish, with a tablespoonful of peas and just one small potato, followed by an apple.

- Your lunchtime meal should also be small. For most people this would mean around 400 calories.

- The same goes for breakfast - 400-500 calories max.

- Avoid processed meals.

- It is normal during the food reintroduction phase for your weight to rise by around two pounds (0.9kg) because you will gain some water as your body balances itself.

By reintroducing food in this graduated way, our volunteers found the transition back to normal eating to be much less troublesome. What they also learned was that there was an opportunity here: eight weeks of eating just a packet for each meal had created a blank slate on which to write new dietary habits. And when they had to fix small meals of 400–500 calories, they tended to rethink the kind of food they would eat.

How to do it – Step 3

By this stage you should feel very proud of yourself. You will have lost a substantial amount of weight. You will hopefully have achieved remission of your type 2 diabetes, and you will be feeling dramatically better, both in mind and body. You will feel more energetic, confident, motivated. Welcome to the beginning of your new life! From now on, you are aiming for a fairly normal pattern of eating which is sustainable for ever – without your regaining weight. And of course drinking alcohol if you wish.

Perhaps it would be safer to call it the 'new normal'. While you can now enjoy eating with family and friends again, and even enjoy the occasional party or special indulgence, if you want to keep the weight off you must avoid slipping back into your old ways and habits.

Stick with these rules of thumb and you will be fine:

- As a rough guide, you will need to eat only three quarters of the amount that you used to eat. So if you ate about 2,400 calories per day before, now it should be about 1,800 calories.

- Write down your weight each week. This is essential. Your weighing scales will tell it how it is. Day to day, your weight may fluctuate. But week to week, if you see steadily rising numbers, you are eating – or maybe drinking – too much. If so, figure out the best way to consume less food or alcohol.

- Try to be more active from day to day. This has to be built into the routine of life and not be something that requires a decision. Get into the habit of walking rather than driving. Always take the stairs, not the lift. Are there any particular activities that would encourage you to be active for longer, most days? If it is your thing, go dancing or get back to badminton. Is there a local 5-a-side league? Remember, the best form of exercise is the one that you enjoy.

- If your weight rises by half a stone (3kg) above target, take immediate action. Recognise the writing on the wall without delay. You need either to go back to the liquid formula diet for a few weeks, or drastically decrease your daily intake of food. Ask yourself whether your usual amount of alcohol is the problem. Whatever you do, don't abandon all the hard work you have put in to regain your health. Think back to why you took action in the first place (read what you wrote down at the time). In a recent big study we conducted in General Practice, rescue plans were needed by one person in two. Weight regain is not necessarily failure. Life will have its ups and downs. Just make sure it is only a temporary blip.

- Don't snack. Ideally, the intensive period of dieting will have changed some of your habits. But if everyone around you is snacking in front of the television it will be hard. Try to avoid any pastime in which your hands are apt to move subconsciously and continuously between packet and mouth. Distract yourself. Find something else to do. Drink water! Sit on your hands!

- Take pride in your written record of weekly weight loss. Enjoy the fact that you can say 'I'm the same weight as I was at the age of [25?] and have been for a year.' And that those last couple of words will eventually become ...'five years'...'ten years' ...'20 years'.

- And, finally, ensure that life is enjoyable. Yes, total food and drink needs to be limited to whatever allows your weight to stay steady, but this must not become a daily burden. It is not the one-off blow-out, but the everyday background intake that is important.

So party, but pay back. You can now join in celebrating the big events of life – anniversaries, birthdays, family occasions – indeed you must! But then you must recognise the need to eat less for a week after these occasions and ensure that your weight goes back to your target level. How will you do this? Well, you might have half-sized portions at one meal each day for a week. Or, if intermittent fasting suits, you might have one day of eating very little. Once again, you need to have a plan ready to put into action.

Previous failure losing weight does not mean failure with this programme

In our studies, a team of psychologists interviewed people to find out what had helped them lose weight and then keep their weight steady, and also to identify what were the main barriers to success. Before the study, many of these people had tried and failed to lose weight. One of the main reasons for this was the slow rate of their weight loss – over a long time trying to stick with it, boredom had set in. Or they had found that the amount of food eaten with friends or family was difficult to change. Nagging hunger had often been a problem on their previous diets, and they had disliked the daily food restriction necessary to continue losing weight. By contrast, most people in our studies thought the 1–2–3 approach was good, both for its speed and because they had felt so well during the low-calorie phase. They also said that ongoing support from their general practice nurse or dietitian was useful in prompting action if their weight started to edge upwards. Overall, they said, the 1–2–3 approach worked because the defined goals of each stage were humanly possible. Also, the early wins increased their motivation to succeed.

The longer follow-up trial, still ongoing, called DiRECT, is showing us that weight regain remains a challenge. There are no easy answers. Our best general advice is stick with it! Without doubt there will be some difficult moments, but overcome these and you will feel hugely empowered. For many of us, it's about suppressing that voice of self-sabotage in the head. As one of our early volunteers told us, 'I was so frazzled one day that I went up to the desk and there were some chocolates right in front of us [me] and I was so tempted to have one but I walked away from them. I have to say I walked up to the tin and lifted the lid three times but each time I just walked away from it because I thought no, because that would have felt like I had given in and I didn't want to do that.' (Woman, aged 35 years, 18 months since diagnosis).

Changing habits

A lot of what we do every day, we do rather automatically. Our actions are determined to a large extent by habit and also by a tendency to do the same as others around us. Before and during your diet it is worth trying to identify particular environmental influences and behaviours that might need to be changed. Our research team have compiled some useful tips for you to think about:

- **Avoidance.** Identify situations of maximum pressure to conform with social eating

- **Distraction.** Have a list of things that you need to do. Mending, fixing, phoning – all those things that may be difficult to bring to mind at the critical moment, but which, if stuck as a to-do list on the fridge, can provide useful distractions. Add to the list: 'Write to MP to remind him/her of the importance of legislating against the advertisement and promotion of high-calorie convenience food '.

- **Drinking water.** Tap water is cheap and good for you! Keep a large jug in the fridge. Drinking a pint of water fills the stomach and occupies the mind during moments of temptation. Fizzy water or flavoured waters with zero calories are also an option to have in the fridge.

- **Removal.** Banish the wrong sort of food from your environment. Your cupboards will ideally be a biscuit-, crisp-, cake-, chocolate-free zone.

- **Reminders.** Keep yourself in touch with your goals. Do write down why you wanted to escape from diabetes in the first place. This can be just a few words on the first page of your diary or on your phone. Perhaps: 1. Not wanting to suffer like Dad. 2. Not to have an upset stomach from those tablets. 3. Wanting not to worry about eyesight or feet or heart. 4. To stop feeling generally unhealthy. It really is worth revisiting your initial motivation for losing weight every now and then – as, however firm our resolve when we embark on a process of change, time will inevitably cause it to fade.

- **Being open with others.** Your family will already be well aware of the reasons why they should not offer you biscuits with your coffee. Hopefully, you can also be entirely open with colleagues and friends about your aim to stay healthy. Just say 'I

> have to watch my weight to stop diabetes
> coming back, so please don't offer me
> things to eat.'

As we have seen, type 2 diabetes is really a case of chronic food poisoning. It is true that not everyone is as susceptible to this food poisoning as you are – and your explanations should not be seen as preaching to family and friends – but everyone can benefit from knowing the fact that body weight should not rise during adult life.

Frequently asked questions

I have been told I have pre-diabetes – what should I do?
Get started on the 1–2–3. By losing approximately one and a half stone (9.5kg), or 10% or your weight if you are less than 12 and a half stone (80kg), you will almost certainly return to normal. You will boost your chance of remaining healthy and enjoying life to the full.

This is the best time to act! At the moment standard medical advice, after a warning blood test, is to come back for another test in a year's time. But my advice is not to hang around when that chap in a hood carrying a scythe comes into view.

Why should I lose weight quickly?
The effect of removing excess fat from inside the liver and

then the pancreas is the same whether weight loss happens over two months or 12 months. The reason for losing the weight fast is that it is easier.

Is it dangerous to lose weight quickly?

No. This is an old idea which unfortunately is still often repeated despite having been disproved. Decreasing food intake to around 800 calories per day for a two-month period has big advantages. Once the diet is underway, you are unlikely to feel very hungry. A second major advantage is that you start feeling so much better within a short period of time that you will want to keep going.

In the first week of a 600–800 calorie diet, the average weight loss is half a stone (3kg); and during the whole eight weeks it is about two and a half stone (15kg). This is a lot! But it should not alarm you: the hard evidence is that for anyone who has increased their weight enough to develop type 2 diabetes, losing the extra weight rapidly and then eating less long term is of *huge* benefit to health. In our overfed society, fasting is not likely to be dangerous, but eating certainly is!

If you have any other health condition, it is always a good idea to discuss with your doctor in advance. If you are on tablets for diabetes or high blood pressure it is very important to do this. Most doctors have now heard about the new findings regarding losing weight effectively.

Can I use a milk diet?

Ideally, you would use the liquid formula packets which provide complete nutrition. But if there is some reason why you cannot, then yes, a milk-based diet (two litres of semi-skimmed milk per day, or about three and a half pints) is both inexpensive and feasible. It will be important to take a multivitamin tablet daily. A portion of non-starchy vegetables should also be included – both to have something to chew on and to provide some roughage.

Why can't I drink alcohol during Step 1?

Because alcohol is best described as liquid fat. Indeed it contains almost as many calories as fat. Alcoholic drinks contain far more calories than is generally realised – around 200 in a pint of beer and about the same in a home-poured glass of wine. It is easier for most people just to to refuse any alcohol-containing drink during Step 1. However, one of our most successful research participants insisted on having a glass of red wine every Friday evening. It was a small glass, and it was sipped very slowly and not refilled. The acid test is whether you are achieving enough weight loss. So provided that you lose around half a stone in the first week and around four pounds each week after that, a glass of wine may be fine. Beer would be problematic given that it is so highly calorific.

Why do I feel cold?

Some people do feel cold all the time while losing weight. It is unlikely that this is due to thinning of the insulating layer of fat under the skin, since feeling cold can come on very soon after starting to lose weight. Feeling cold is more likely to be caused by the smaller amounts of heat generated by the body when it does not have to deal with so much food. The only thing you can do is to wrap up warmly (thermal vest?). It is certainly preferable to feeling too heavy and too sweaty.

If my hair thins will it regrow?

This is rare, but the answer is yes – in time. A few people do notice hair thinning after weight loss. In fact, lots of things (exams, pregnancy, family illness) can cause the growth cycle of all the hairs to become synchronised. Normally, around 70 hairs per day fall out as they come to the end of their growth cycle. If one cycle of growth falls into step with another, several hundred will fall out every day – but only for a limited period. Don't worry: your hair will grow back. Of course, this advice does not apply if the hair loss is due to a different cause.

What do I do if I get constipated?

There are people who, despite chomping through a large plate of lettuce, celery, peppers and tomatoes every single day, find that they are still constipated while dieting. What to do? The simplest thing is to take a medicine that will bulk up your bowel movements. Fybogel is one that can be bought from chemists or supermarkets. But if the problem persists do consult your own doctor.

Can weight loss cause gallstones?

A low-calorie diet will make gallstones smaller. Oddly, this can on rare occasions cause problems, as the smaller gallstones can then find their way from the gall bladder into the tube that carries the digestive juices into the gut and possibly get stuck there, causing pain. In people with type 2 diabetes, gallstones are very common – affecting around one person in five – so one might assume that they would be at higher risk of a stone becoming troublesome during weight loss. But in our biggest research study, only one person had gall bladder trouble out of the 149 who had lost weight during the study. This is about the same number that would be expected in any group of people with type 2 diabetes having usual treatment. So, although there is a small risk of having a biliary attack as gallstones get smaller, there is a chance of this anyway in the future by doing nothing.

Can I change where the fat disappears from?

Sometimes it seems as though the fat is dropping away

from all the wrong places. Sadly, we have no way of affecting this. In fact, it often amazes me that even now, with our detailed knowledge about so much, we have no idea what determines where fat is stored in any one person's body. What controls this? What stops it being heaped together in a hump somewhere? Apart from the obvious effect of sex hormones on the distribution of some parts of the fat layer in a typically female or male pattern, we have no idea.

Can I avoid looking puny after weight loss?

This might sound an odd question, given that most people today would like to look slim and fit. But this is a question we are often asked by people in important jobs. There was a time in the UK when most company directors, civic mayors and leaders would be large, imposing people. That is less the case today. In other cultures, being impressively large is of greater importance. Take a look at some of the top people elsewhere in the world: you might spot that many of them are large. What can you do about no longer looking so impressive after weight loss? The best way is to lift weights regularly to build up the neck and shoulder muscles. And to have self-confidence. Shoulders back and chin up. Do the James Bond walk! You don't need extra weight to give the impression of clout.

You can find much more on both the science and the practice of the 1–2–3 approach on our website – https://go.ncl.ac.uk/diabetes-reversal and in my book *Life Without Diabetes* which also gives a full explanation of type 2 diabetes and what happens inside your body during the return to normal health.

Quick read

- Losing weight rapidly is easier for most people than a long drawn-out effort.

- Eight weeks on a low-calorie diet is not easy, but is far more doable than you would expect.

- The hardest part is keeping the weight steady into the future, but there are a few key lifestyle changes that can really help.

- It's all about positive reinforcement: the longer you stay slim, the more motivated you will feel to keep the weight off.

Chapter 7

Enjoying life and staying diabetes-free

Having succeeded in getting your weight down, you will be feeling better than you have for years, ready to embrace life with renewed vigour and confidence. And so you should. But do not relax too much! From now on, there is a simple bottom line – you must avoid weight regain. You will not be able to return to eating the amount you used to regard as normal.

Golden principles for a life without diabetes:

1. Only eat at meal times. Not between meals.
2. Don't do other things while eating. If you eat while reading, working or watching television, far more slips down than you notice.

3. Avoid ready meals and fast foods – they usually contain added sugar and tend to leave you feeling hungry. There are plenty of easy meals made with fresh ingredients that can be microwaved in minutes.

4. Avoid sweetened drinks of all kinds (except the ones that contain zero calories).

5. Party, but pay back. Enjoy that special occasion. Life is for living. But after you've had your fun, the next week is crucial. For the next seven days you must cut back on what you eat.

6. Regular physical activity – day by day, year by year – is important. But remember the balance between eating and physical activity is very one-sided: a couple of extra mouthfuls of food can easily cancel out the effects of half an hour of exercise.

What happens to your body after weight loss

Big animals need more food than small animals. If you have lost weight, you have a smaller body to keep alive, so you need less food.

This is sometimes dressed up in scientific language – 'your metabolic rate has decreased'. But that makes it sound mysterious and difficult to fight. The real problem is habit – a very human problem. Most of our lives run on autopilot. It would be exhausting to make new decisions every minute of the day. Therefore we easily slip back into old habits.

Think about how you eat: when do you find yourself eating? And with whom? How much do you usually put on your plate? How often do you cook fresh foods rather than using ready meals? It is vital to know your own eating habits if you are going to make effective changes.

Troubleshooting

There are many potential reasons why you might begin to regain weight. Below I have listed some of the most obvious ones, and some advice on how to head them off before too much damage is done.

1. Difficult life events

One of the commonest ways of being blown off course is when something bad happens. I have seen this countless times in my patients: they are doing fine, maintaining a reasonably steady weight, and then there is an illness in the family or trouble at work, or some other adverse event and everything goes to pot. Life does not run smoothly all the time. The Covid-19 lockdowns were difficult for many people for instance. Naturally, if you have a problem or worry, it fills your mind. And, in the meantime, all that business of avoiding old habits and being careful about food tends to fade into the background. Yes, it still seems important, but it is no longer at the forefront.

There is a key message to be taken from this. You need to be prepared for how you are going to manage when life gets tough. Being aware is a good start, but you should have a rescue plan at the ready. It is too late to think about ordering a life belt when you are already in the water.

This is one of the clearest lessons we learned from our research. Rescue plans had to be lined up in advance. If someone gained more than half a stone in weight, we encouraged them to go back onto a low-calorie liquid formula diet to shed the extra weight as soon as possible. But any way of severely cutting back the amount you eat can be successful. You just need to do it.

Not recognising that life events occur, and that the stress of these makes us likely to regain weight, is the reason why so many of us find our weight rising unchecked over the years.

2. The slow creep upwards

A second pattern of weight regain is the gradual increase – for no apparent reason. It's not that there has been any change in your routine, there has not been a series of big parties to contend with, just somehow week on week, month on month, you are slowly gaining pounds. This means only one thing: you are taking in more food or drink than you really need. Sorting this out requires an honest look at what is happening.

- Think about your food habits: whether you are eating between meals; or simply putting too much on your plate. By hook or by crook, these behaviours have to be tackled.

- What about alcohol? You may have to decide that you can only have beer, wine or spirits at weekends, or you need to substitute some of them with zero-calorie drinks. Perhaps you struggle with the social pressure of buying rounds. That is why it is so important to enlist the help of your friends. Real friends don't mind you having a pint of Coke zero or a low-calorie bitter lemon.

- Is there a hidden problem that is working at your subconscious? Mild stress at work? It may be nothing new, but perhaps it is getting to you more than you realise. It is important to recognise this, as the worry of it will chronically divert your efforts away from keeping your weight steady.

3. Your package holiday!

It is easy to understand how it happens: you have been away from your routine, in a glorious escapist bubble. And, after all, it's only once a year…But unfortunately having pre-paid food in limitless quantities is a sure recipe for putting on weight. Sometimes holiday weight gain can be huge in a short time.

On your return home you must take urgent action: type 2 diabetes is ready to spring its trap. So it's back to a few weeks of liquid meals, drastically reduced portions – whatever it takes.

4. Medicines

Steroids cause weight gain. Not those 'anabolic steroids' which hit the headlines as drugs misused by some athletes or bodybuilders. We are talking about the vital medical steroids prescribed by doctors as treatment for some serious illnesses. These drugs have a major effect on appetite. There is no easy answer to this powerful, unwanted effect. But fortunately, few people require high doses of steroids for months on end, and so once the medical problem has gone away, a few weeks of weight loss is needed.

Some drugs used to treat type 2 diabetes can cause weight gain. Insulin can do this. So can some kinds of tablets – sulfonylureas (such as gliclazide) and TZDs (such as pioglitazone). Talk to your doctor if you are taking tablets and want to try to get rid of your diabetes – never stop taking them without discussing it first.

Although, as I mentioned above, not all doctors are yet completely up to speed on diabetes reversal, I'm delighted to say that our research has been put to widespread use much more rapidly than many other medical discoveries. Indeed, an NHS trial is currently underway in the UK based on the 1–2–3 approach outlined in this book. The programme is being rolled out in a bid to find the most effective way of providing the necessary advice and support for people at minimum cost to the NHS.

Low fat, low carb… Is there really a best way?

Magazine and newspapers are full of 'diets'. Lots of them. Diets with fancy names. But there is no one diet that suits everyone.

The basics of what you need from food were sorted out over a century ago. Those basics remain just the same today:

1. The body needs a certain amount of energy, and you get this from fat, carbohydrate or protein.
2. Protein and some fats are essential, but only in modest amounts.

3. We need vitamins – in tiny amounts. If you eat a reasonable variety of foods, true vitamin deficiency is relatively unlikely. Don't fall for the advertising gimmick of cereal manufacturers!

4. We need enough minerals, especially iron.

5. To function properly, our bowels need fibre from vegetables.

These basics are really simple. And the truth is that when it comes to diets there is no one supreme 'healthy diet'. As I mentioned earlier, individuals have their own food preferences, and cultures across the world eat differently.

However, there is one respect in which you call the shots. That is regarding the amount of food you eat. It is wrong to say that you are what you eat – you are *how much* you eat.

If your weight has gone up by more than a small amount since your mid twenties, then your diet has not been healthy. Excess fat inside your body carries far more risk to health than does the kind of food you consume.

There are a number of approaches that might help you limit your overall calorie intake. I outline these in the next few pages – while also trying to explode a few myths that have grown up regarding food in recent decades. If you are not sure yet which type of diet is best for you, perhaps try those that appeal to you one by one. Only you can judge what works for you.

Myths about food: No .1

Red meat is dangerous!

My colleague Professor Michael Roden, who is Director of the German Diabetes Research Centre in Dusseldorf, found that people who ate a lot of red meat were more insulin-resistant than those who did not. Almost always, the result of this kind of big study is taken at face value, and beliefs about the evils of red meat spread.

But Michael is an all-round scientist, so he went on to find out whether red meat really 'caused' the trouble – or whether it was just guilty by association. And sure enough he found that when one group of people deliberately ate lots of red meat and another deliberately ate none, there was absolutely no effect on insulin resistance. It was simply that eating lots of red meat is *associated* with eating a lot, full stop. It is just a marker for eating a lot of food – it does not itself cause insulin resistance.

And, to clear up another misapprehension: although insulin resistance leads to increased risk of heart disease and cancers, there is no evidence that eating red meat actually causes heart disease or cancer, and most certainly not if you are maintaining a weight that is healthy for you.

Had it not been for proper scientific work focusing on this precise question, the myths surrounding red meat would have persisted.

Low carb?

Carbohydrates make up around half the calories in the average British diet. Most other European countries eat less (43–45%). At the same time, the UK is the Fat Man of Europe. This statistic is far from proof of cause but it does suggest that moderately limiting carbohydrates (such as sugar) can help with long-term weight control.

Even so, there is a problem in talking about low-carb diets, as different people mean different things by the term. How low is low?

At the extreme, there are very low-carbohydrate diets on which you would eat no bread, potato, pasta or rice at all. They are sometimes called 'keto' diets. Ignore the fancy names which suggest some kind of magic; these diets can achieve weight loss, although there are some health risks attached to them.

For most people, though, 'low carb' would mean

eating a modest amount of starchy vegetables and fruit (a small potato, carrots, avocado and an apple or pear), perhaps with a portion of rice or a slice of bread each day. This is a perfectly sensible way to proceed: everything in moderation! And it has the advantage of being something you can do when eating with other people. When eating out, you simply put most of the potato/rice/pasta to the side and leave it untouched (difficult for people who have been brought up to 'clear your plate' – such an ingrained notion from the past).

It may suit some people to use carbohydrate restriction at a single meal. Perhaps none in your evening meal? Or decide no bread or wraps at lunchtime?

The key thing is to be aware of the hidden carbs in processed food and ready meals which often have sugar added. Try and cook from scratch whenever you can. It doesn't need to be complicated: a one-pan meal of fried bacon, broccoli, mushrooms and tomatoes is delicious and can be rustled up in minutes.

And, remember, no fruit juices and smoothies! All these contain concentrated carbohydrate as sugar, and this includes the ones misleadingly labelled 'no added sugar'. Sugar is sugar, whether grown in a field or made in a factory.

Breakfast cereals are out. Huge amounts of money are spent trying to make you believe they are 'healthy' but they are not a good idea. Why not go to work on an egg?

Lunch at work? You don't have to rely on a sandwich or a wrap. Take a slice of cheese, an apple and some nuts – no prep required and easy to carry.

Myths about food: No 2

Eggs are bad for you!

Eggs contain cholesterol. So when high levels of cholesterol were found to be a risk factor for heart attacks, foods containing cholesterol were assumed to be bad for the heart.

Then the rumour mill started. Don't eat more than one egg per day! Better still, avoid all eggs! Even doctors believed it was true. After all, it seemed obvious. Cholesterol 'causes' heart attacks and eggs contain cholesterol.

But before jumping to conclusions, we need to take a step back and ask a couple of questions:

'Does cholesterol itself cause heart attacks?' We know that blood cholesterol is *higher in people with a higher risk* of heart attacks – but this does not prove that it actually causes heart attacks.

'Does eating eggs raise our cholesterol levels?' The simple answer is 'No'.

It is true that people who eat more than they need tend to eat more eggs and also have higher cholesterol. But, as with red meat, it is eating too much that is the likely cause of trouble. It has nothing to do with the cholesterol content of eggs.

Cholesterol is vital for life and your body makes a lot of it every day. It is needed by all the cells of the body and you would fall apart without it. In comparison with the amount of cholesterol you make naturally for yourself, the contribution of an egg or two is very small.

Beware of any new stories 'proving' that eggs are bad for you. They are likely to be merely repeating the same old mistake.

Mediterranean?

The 'Mediterranean' diet is great – provided you find it enjoyable and can build it into your life. It is based on eating lots of vegetables, olive oil and meats or cheeses, and not very much bread/pasta etc.

There are lots of recipe books on this kind of diet, although you don't need to follow complicated recipes to take a Med-style approach to eating: a simple meal of grilled chicken or fish and lots of vegetables would fit the bill very well. That said, this is a diet which probably needs a little more planning than, say, just cutting back on the amounts you eat or simply missing some foods out.

Intermittent fasting?

The '5:2' diet is very popular. It involves eating normally on five days of the week andeating very little on the other two. Then, after achieving the weight loss you want, you carry on with a 6:1 approach, where one day per week is a fasting day with minimal food. Although some people find they cannot get on with this, it suits others very well indeed, especially when couples follow the regime together.

One variation of intermittent fasting is simply to miss out one meal altogether every day. For those people who do not particularly like eating breakfast, and can get used to not eating until lunchtime, this approach is ideal. There is no truth whatever in the catch phrase 'breakfast is the most important meal of the day' (see the box below).

Or you could try 'timed fasting' – where you eat only within a certain time window each day. For instance, you could eat normally from 12 noon until 8pm, but nothing outside that window of time. Or decide you are going to eat nothing before 2pm, or nothing after 6pm. Just now there is no proof that this keeps weight down in the long term, but if it suits you and your family and friends, go for it. Your weighing scales will tell you if it is working.

Myths about food: No. 3

'Breakfast is the most important meal of the day'

This catch phrase is so often repeated that it is rarely questioned. But it is simply an advertising slogan invented by the breakfast cereal industry.

What is not so well advertised is that the industry pays for a steady stream of studies every year to maintain the myth. These studies are carefully designed to give only one answer - that people who eat breakfast tend to be slimmer than those who skip it. Which is quite different from testing whether overweight people who start eating breakfast will become slimmer! Of course they would not. There are a whole host of reasons why breakfast eaters tend to be slimmer. For example, if you satisfy your hunger with something at breakfast time you are less likely to end up snacking on a high-sugar, high-fat snack during the morning.

For people who can't function without breakfast, it is far better that they eat before leaving the house. A boiled egg, maybe, or a bowl of porridge. But if you would prefer just to have a cup of coffee on waking, well-designed studies show that you will eat less each day - by avoiding that unwanted breakfast-time meal.

Individuals are individuals, and the myth of 'breakfast is mandatory' needs to be consigned to history.

Low fat?

A low-fat diet to lose weight sounds so effective. Fats contain the most calories. This is stretched to assume that it is best to limit your fat consumption. However, fat can make food taste better, and if you remove too much of it, you end up with a rather grim, dry mouthful, which is unlikely to prove a sustainable way of eating. Low-fat diets can keep weight down but many people find it difficult to stick to them in the long term.

Beware foods sold as 'low-fat'. They often have added sugar or other ingredients to make them taste better. They are rarely very low in calories. And they may not satisfy your appetite for long.

Myths about food: No. 4

Killer fat!

In the 1960s, a study comparing rates of heart disease in different countries found that it was commoner in the richer ones. No surprise there, because in affluent countries people could afford to have a lot of food. But the study just reported that the more fat that was eaten the more heart attacks occurred. That caused the US government to advise that fat consumption should be decreased. Incredibly, they were heavily influenced by the fact that President Eisenhower had just suffered a heart attack, and 'something had to be done'.

The snag was that lots of information from the study had not been considered, especially that people in richer countries could afford to eat more and therefore put on a lot more weight.

Big problems occur when a scientific misconception is adopted and propagated in health policy by governments. Even when governments get it wrong, the error tends to become the accepted norm - sometimes internationally.

Since that 1960s study, many newer studies have shown that fat itself is not bad for you - simply that, if you eat a lot of fat, you are likely to be eating too much overall.

> For some people, a moderately high-fat, lower-carbohydrate diet is the easiest way to avoid overeating as, for them, the fat is very satisfying. That is fine, and if this helps you lose weight and keep it off - go for it. Remember, it is the total amount of food that determines the risk of weight gain in the long term, and it is the weight gain that increases the risk to health.

So there you have it: four different approaches to weight loss. There is only one way to find out if a particular way of eating is good for you. Suck it and see! You may really lock onto a low-carb approach. Great. You may do well on an intermittent fasting approach. Excellent. Discover what really suits you for long-term health and happiness.

A last word on alcohol

I certainly wouldn't advocate a total ban on alcohol. For many people it is a source of much enjoyment and can be built into a way of life consistent with keeping weight steady. However, the increased dependency on alcohol that has happened during the Covid-19 pandemic lockdowns is worrying. Don't allow yourself to drift into needing alcohol as that will certainly *prevent* you from enjoying life to the full.

Everything depends on quantity. An evening out with a large glass of wine (or pint of beer) followed by zero calorie drinks will bless you with around 200 calories. Not bad, provided it is not every night. But if five glasses of wine or five pints have slipped down, that adds 1,000 calories to your daily intake. And that could add almost a quarter of a pound of fat (100g) to your body. In just one heavy night out.

No wonder an expanding waistline is sometimes referred to as a 'beer-belly'.

The basic message on alcohol is to enjoy it if you like. But only as long as you are honest with yourself about how you are consuming and it does not affect your weight in the long term.

Why do we overeat?

Many of us browse around to find something to eat when we are a little bored. Then before long, one snack between breakfast and lunch is joined by another mid-afternoon and another before bed...

Why do we do this? Over 200,000 years of human evolution we have had to search out available food as the number one priority. There would often be periods of food scarcity, which might be due to natural disasters or social upheavals. Everyone had to make hay while the sun shone. Those who were best at eating as much as was available would survive the next cycle of crop failure or the lack of success hunting. They were better at survival, full stop. Poorly nourished people are less fertile – just look at old fertility symbols and you will see that they are all very well rounded. If you don't eat well, you risk not passing on your genes.

However, the people who have the biggest appetites and seek out food most successfully have been rudely wrong-footed in today's world. Even the poorest in our society can obtain excess things to eat. And this is not good news. In our present environment, the people who would have been best at surviving bad times have become disadvantaged.

Continuing the species, of course, is an absolute necessity. And so, as a result of evolution, we have developed clever mechanisms to remind us to eat. Hormones acting on the brain encourage us to find food and this promotes the chances of survival. On the other hand, we have evolved absolutely no mechanism whatsoever to prevent over-accumulation of fat in the body. To make it worse, we can still feel hungry, even though the body may be groaning under the influence of excess fat.

Overall, if you are a person who has tended to

increase in weight since the age of 21 years, then you should be proud of your genes – but look out. You are living not in an environment of food scarcity but in one where you have to curb your eating habits. Just remember: your body is designed to work just fine without any food for quite long periods. The gap between lunch and dinner is only a few hours. Why would you voluntarily push calories into your mouth between meals? Take a look in your cupboards. Check there are no biscuits, no crisps, no cakes, no chocolate, no sweets.

How about your fridge? Remember that jug of tap water (so that if you feel desperately peckish, you can drink a pint of cold, refreshing water). Certainly, your fridge should never contain fruit juice or fruit smoothies. These dangerous calorie bombs slip down too easily and do not satisfy hunger. Contrary to the claims of seductive advertisements, there is nothing healthy about them.

Time for a new foodrobe!

Lucia, one of our psychology team, coined a nice word. She studied how our volunteers coped with getting back to normal eating, after losing weight. And she found that, for most of them, getting used to cooking and eating ordinary foods again was more difficult than losing weight. It was a challenge to know which foods to buy and which to avoid. So Lucia invented the new word 'foodrobe'. And, as in a wardrobe, where you put the clothes you buy, she encouraged our volunteers to think about building up a new foodrobe to suit their lives going forwards – one with no easy snacks to tempt them, no sugary drinks, no commercial ready meals; just good honest food to be prepared for mealtimes.

Getting around

The best chance you have of being the same weight in ten years' time is by building in more physical activity every day. As long as – and this is crucial – you do not take this as a cue to eat more. Those vending machines or low shelves positioned for maximum temptation? Walk straight past them.

The 'best' activity is the one you enjoy: walking, gardening, dancing, aerobics, table tennis, even running. The point is to build a reasonable level of physical activity into each day. How? Make it part of getting where you have to go. For instance, people living in London walk the furthest in the UK, simply because the majority of them cannot park anywhere near their place of work. People living in London also have the lowest average BMI in the UK. Maybe this is because they do so much walking.

Remember, absolutely anywhere is within walking

distance – if you have the time. However, in practice, for longer distances, cycling can be good – anything other than sitting in a car or on a bus.

A little help from my friends

The Beatles immortalised the idea of 'getting by with a little help from my friends' – and it strikes a chord. Some help from your friends can be so important in coping with the everyday problems of life. When unpredictable events upset your day or equilibrium, your best intentions may be tested and you may not be able to pick yourself up.

Who can help? Over to you. It could be your spouse, partner, friend, healthcare professional, muse, barber/hairdresser – the list of possibilities is endless.

I learned in our very first study of reversing type 2 diabetes that successfully losing weight wasn't just up to the individual. One big predictor of success was the 'significant other'. The partner, spouse, relative or friend… And I found this often proved to be a two-way street, as the other person often lost weight too. Overall, this is a clear sign that the home environment has changed, with cupboards temptation-free.

We can't stop life's stresses happening. But it is possible derailing us. Get a little help from your friends.

And, finally, speak out!

The main focus of this book is of course you – your bid to change your life and restore yourself to full health and wellbeing. But ultimately good health is also a public health story, one that impacts on every one of us.

In the UK, the NHS spends an estimated £6.1 billion annually (2014–2015 figures) on treating obesity, and a further £10 billion on type 2 diabetes. We spend more each year on the treatment of obesity and diabetes than we do on the police, fire service and judicial system combined. Ouch. Tax payers need to know this.

We now have a generation of children who are already too heavy at the start of adult life. Type 2 diabetes is coming on at younger and younger ages. This is extremely concerning as the disease is far more dangerous in younger people.

As I have explained, the diabetes crisis is not caused by greedy, lazy people. It is largely caused by the food-laden environment in which we live. And we desperately need legal regulation regarding the sale of harmful foods.

You'd think stricter controls on the sale and promotion of calorie-heavy foods would be a no-brainer. Yet whenever this is proposed, well-meaning voices – and some less well-meaning – are raised against it. A similar chorus of loud voices spoke out against compulsory use of seat belts and motorcycle helmets, and against legislation on smoking. You don't hear those same voices lamenting the dramatic fall in deaths of parents, brothers and sisters that followed legislation on each of these once-controversial matters.

Action is so desperately needed. Clear calorie labelling, limiting fast-food outlets close to schools, a reduction in the sugar content of snacks and processed foods, and limiting of mega-size or two-for-one bargains would all be excellent first steps.

How to get this done? Well, one simple thing you can do, if you have succeeded in turning your life around and have escaped from diabetes and kept it away, is to speak out! Use social media, call in to radio programmes, write letters to papers – use any means to get the wider message across. Type 2 diabetes is not a hopeless condition; and no one person's situation is hopeless. The more you can provide real-life stories to help balance out the unregulated propaganda from the food industry the better.

My challenge to you is to help make things better for our children.

Quick read

- Once in remission, type 2 diabetes will stay away if you keep your weight steady

- The key is to find a way to live happily while eating only around three quarters of the amount you used to

- Building walking or other activity into everyday life can help you do this

- Different patterns of eating suit different people – no one diet suits everyone!

- Moderate carbohydrate limitation may be simplest for some people; others are best suited to a Mediterranean (+ low-carb) pattern of eating, and/or intermittent fasting

- Recognising alcohol as liquid fat is important to keep calories down

- The diabetes epidemic is due to our environment, not the result of a sudden increase in greed and sloth

- Slow action by law-makers is costing tax payers billions of pounds each year in the costs of treating type 2 diabetes and its associated problems

- National regulation of foods will be essential to make an impact on the epidemic.

Acknowledgements

Behind every leap forward in medical knowledge is a story about people. I am hugely grateful to the people behind what I have to say in this book. They include the volunteers who gave up time – and blood – to help with the research, my own patients over more than four decades, and the doctors and scientists who have worked with me. Research work needs money, and I am very grateful to Diabetes UK, the charity that provided grants to do the research leading to the breakthroughs described in this book.

I have no commercial ties. I serve on a UK government working group assessing the published evidence about low carbohydrate diets. The views expressed in this book are personal and not those of the committee.

This work would not have been possible without long hours of absence from family – usually absent in body, but frequently absent in mind. I am so grateful for the very longstanding forbearance and support of Aileen, my wife, and sons James, Donald, Alasdair and Duncan.

Further reading

Life Without Diabetes by Roy Taylor (Short Books).

This book goes into more detail about how the body deals with food and how type 2 diabetes develops.

Website: https://go.ncl.ac.uk/diabetes-reversal

This website includes the basic information on how to reverse type 2 diabetes and provides more detail about the science behind *Your Simple Guide to Reversing Type 2 Diabetes*.

Index

obesity 25
  financial cost of 138
  growth (UK) 60–1
  type 2 diabetes and 26–7,
    46, 67
  see also overeating; weight
    gain
openness 107–8
Optifast 95
  overeating 131–2, 133–5
  mindlessly 62–3
  see also weight gain

package holidays 120
pancreas 19, 29
  fat and 47–8
  functions of 50
  importance of 42–3
  location of 48–9, 50
  secret life of 48–51
  shrinkage of 51, 52
  size of 51–3
  storage of fat in 45
personal fat threshold 54–68,
    76, 78
  ethnic groups 67–8
  meaning of 66
  rapid weight loss 75–6
physical activity *see* exercise
Pima Indians 26
population (UK) 59–62
pre-diabetes 27–8, 29, 108
pride 103
processed food 125
protein 44, 93, 95

public health 138
puny appearance 113–14

rapid weight loss *see* step 1
    (1-2-3 diet)
ready meals 45, 116, 125
red meat 123–4
reminders 107
removal, of unhealthy foods 107
rescue plans 118
Roden, Professor Michael 123

sex hormones 113
side effects 31–2, 33
skin infections 21
snacking 103, 115
social occasions 80–1, 104, 116
special meals 97
start-up dinner (step 2) 100
step 1 (1-2-3 diet) 91, 94–9
  advantages 109
  alcohol 110
  feeling good 98–9, 105
  people's thoughts on 98–9
  tips for managing 96–7
step 2 (1-2-3 diet) 91, 99–100
step 3 (1-2-3 diet) 91, 101–4
steroids 120
stress 119
strokes 23, 28
sugar 17, 48
  in food 45
  misleading labelling 125
  releasing of 43
  see also blood sugar levels

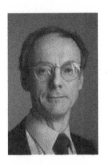

Professor Roy Taylor is Professor of Medicine
and Metabolism at Newcastle University and
Honorary Consultant Physician at Newcastle upon
Tyne Hospitals NHS Foundation Trust. He qualified in
Medicine at the University of Edinburgh. He was visiting
Professor of Medicine at Yale University, USA (1990-91)
where he acquired new MRI methods to look into the
human body. On returning to the UK he raised £5.2
million to establish the Newcastle MR Centre. He also
developed the UK system for screening of diabetic eye
disease and is the author of over 300 scientific papers.